T0067906

Dementia Caregiving
FROM A
Biblical Perspective

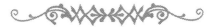

Your Guide for the Journey

DOROTHY GABLE

WESTBOW
PRESS®
A DIVISION OF THOMAS NELSON
& ZONDERVAN

WestBow Press books may be ordered through booksellers or by contacting:

WestBow Press
A Division of Thomas Nelson & Zondervan
1663 Liberty Drive
Bloomington, IN 47403
www.westbowpress.com
1 (866) 928-1240

Interior Image Credit: Jude Gilbert; Lindsay Billington

Scripture quotations are from the ESV® Bible (The Holy Bible, English Standard Version®), copyright © 2001 by Crossway, a publishing ministry of Good News Publishers. Used by permission. All rights reserved.

ISBN: 978-1-9736-7662-1 (sc)
ISBN: 978-1-9736-7664-5 (hc)
ISBN: 978-1-9736-7663-8 (e)

Library of Congress Control Number: 2019915699

Print information available on the last page.

WestBow Press rev. date: 10/23/2019

Contents

Introduction

As I stood just ouftside my mother's room at the Sienna Crest assisted living center, I paused to calm myself. Forcing deep, slow breaths, I felt my heartbeat settle out and my busy mind ramp down.

Mom lay on her left side, the body pillow following the curve of her spine and bent legs. I pulled a chair around and sat down quietly. Her eyes remained closed; her hands, reduced to skin and bones, clutched a large stuffed dog.

I lay my hand on hers and leaned over to place a quick peck on her cheek.

She opened her eyes and smiled, trying to mouth some words. I knew what she was trying to say, what she always said when I came to visit her, "I'm so glad you're here."

"Hello, Mom. I love you," I said softly in her ear.

After living with dementia for several years, Mom was in her final stretch and close to her last days on earth.

I sat back in the chair and turned my head. I had prayed God would spare her from going through the final stages and let her die peacefully in her sleep. I had waited for the call that never came. Instead, God chose to allow her go through all the stages of dementia.

This short time on earth is a light, momentary affliction—a limited season of sorrow. Our loving God chose my mother's pathway to heaven to go through the dementia journey. He never promised to remove the sorrows, but accompanies us through them. We have a heavenly future waiting for us as we step through death's door.

After my father died, while my three sisters and I helped Mom settle his estate, it became clear to us she could not live on her own. Despite surviving polio, my mother was fairly healthy. She had no heart disease, cancer, pulmonary disease or diabetes. We did not realize her brain was already impaired and in the early stages of dementia. After all, wasn't forgetfulness part of old age? She had just lost her life mate of 50 years, and she could be scatterbrained at times. We all assumed she would grieve, and once she had adjusted, would stabilize.

She just needed a little help and there was room at my house. Mom and Dad had four daughters – Dorothy, Ann, Joan and Louise. I am the oldest, my kids were grown and out of the house, and my job was the standard 40 hours. Before the end of the month after Dad's sudden passing, Mom and her earthly belongings were traveling to my home in Wisconsin. All would be well.

I did not truly understand she had dementia until a few years after she moved to Sienna Crest, a small assisted living facility a short distance from our home. Even though she loved the social stimulation of the close-knit community at her facility, she did not stabilize. Her cognitive abilities continued to erode.

I didn't know the best ways to help her or understand why she acted the way she did. I didn't understand the differences between Alzheimer's and dementia, and the doctor never uttered a diagnosis. Not knowing dementia is a set of symptoms caused by a number of diseases, including Alzheimer's, I thought she had dementia but not Alzheimer's. I didn't realize the Alzheimer's name had become an umbrella term encompassing many diseases causing dementia. I was too busy working full time and going to night school, besides caring for her, to do the research. I merely coped from day to day, eventually figuring out how to relate to her as her world shrank.

As she lost the ability to remember Bible verses, doctrines and, eventually, His name, I found myself questioning the value of her efforts to study and memorize if it's lost at the end. How could I show her honor and respect while taking more and more of the role of caring for her? How do I speak truth to her as she lost grasp of the decade she inhabited? Some days, she asked where my father was, having lost the memory of his death.

After my mother's death, and my husband, Ralph, and I relocated to another city, I began to look for answers. Was Alzheimer's the same as dementia? Why did she forget her husband had died? How was it possible for her to remember something months after it seemed the memory had been lost?

Over time, I decided to write a book for the Christian caregiver to help chart the dementia journey. Understanding how the diseases that cause dementia impact the brain and alter the actions of our loved ones helps us find ways to minister to them. How do we tell her the truth in love when she has become disoriented? Is there value in visiting our loved one if it is likely she will not remember who we are and she will forget the visit moments after we leave? How do we honor our parents when we become their caregivers? Should we sign the forms so she will not be resuscitated if her heart stops? Should we have a feeding tube installed if she can no longer eat?

Walking through dementia's progression in an individual, I will seek to show the way and demonstrate why these symptoms can cause her to act strangely. I will share the lessons my three sisters and I learned in helping our mother live with dementia and prepare for the Lord's coming for her. I will seek to answer: What does dementia do to the person you love? Are they truly gone? How do you relate to her as she changes? What changes can you expect to see and how do you handle them? Most of all, I will seek to share the blessings of God, and the lessons we learned as we helped our mother live out her life and finish her race well.

Part One

UNDERSTANDING DEMENTIA

1

Normal Brain Aging or Dementia?

A few years before my father, Glenn, died due to complications from surgery, Mom told me she thought she was getting Alzheimer's. She would forget to send the usual birthday cards to some family members, while sending multiple cards and checks to others.

Wondering if her difficulties did point to Alzheimer's, I briefly researched the topic on the internet. When I called her a few weeks later, I broached the subject. Embarrassed, Mom said, "Oh, the doctor told me I don't have Alzheimer's. I'm doing fine, just getting older."

I let it drop. At least she did not have Alzheimer's, I told myself. Relief mixed with confusion since she did seem to have some mental lapses. If not Alzheimer's, then what caused them?

While settling the estate after Dad's death, it became clear that Mom could not live alone in their isolated retirement home in north central New York state. Their home had wood heat, experienced frequent snow and ice, and Mom relied on a walker to get around. More than the physical challenges, we also realized she could not mentally handle running her household.

Believing my mother did not have Alzheimer's, I assumed she was just aging and needed a little more attention. However, some of the things she said puzzled me because they had little basis in reality.

Knowing she once had a good memory, I tried to correct her in order to orient her to the truth. This turned into daily corrections leading to awkward silences. I came to realize, when she couldn't find her hearing aids, her explanations of where they could be had little basis in fact. She seemed to live in a different world. She said she did not have Alzheimer's, but I knew something was wrong.

This seemed to go beyond normal aging. Had she always been this absent-minded? Mom would remark, "I feel so dumb. I used to have a good memory." I tried to reassure her, along with myself that everything was OK, but I continued to ponder the possibility of dementia. Is there a difference between normal brain aging, dementia and Alzheimer's disease?

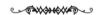

Story Illustrations

To illustrate concepts I will use personal stories from time to time. Some will be drawn from my family's experience with my mother's dementia journey during the time she lived with us, my husband Ralph and myself, and at Sienna Crest, a nearby assisted living facility. While not living close by, my three sisters, Ann, Joan and Louise, helped greatly and visited Mom often.

My mother had Alzheimer's type dementia mixed with vascular cognitive impairment. I will also include stories from others with Alzheimer's disease, Lewy body dementia or frontotemporal dementia. In some stories the names were changed for privacy.

Dementia Definition

When a person has increasing problems with two or more cognitive or mental abilities severe enough to interfere with daily living, she has *dementia*. This general term does not refer to a disease, but to a set of symptoms, just as fever is a symptom caused by many different diseases. Someone's personality can shift or reverse; the ability to remember recent events can erode; a person could lose connection with where she is living or the decade she inhabits; she could forget the order of steps to make coffee, get dressed, or cook a meal; she could lose her ability to analyze, reason, and understand abstract concepts, including numbers. The mind of a person with dementia seems to have fundamentally changed.

Dementia differs from the natural decline in cognitive skills due to aging, or delirium (passing loss of consciousness and/or reality). While some decline occurs with age, this does not lead to loss of abilities to reason, calculate or remember. Structural changes in the brain due to normal brain aging are different from the organic brain damage caused by the diseases that produce dementia symptoms.[1]

Many diseases produce the progressive, terminal form of dementia. The best known is *Alzheimer's disease.* However dementia can also be caused by *vascular cognitive impairment, frontotemporal dementia* (also known as frontotemporal degeneration), or *Lewy body dementia.* These are the four main types of diseases with many variations. Each disease type has its own trajectory and each individual's expression of dementia is unique. No one person has every symptom.

The damage to cells in the brain starts in a few areas and spreads until eventually encompassing most areas. It not only impacts thought processes, emotions, and will, but also the brain's ability to keep the body healthy. With dementia, the increasing cognitive deficits make it impossible to live independently. In the beginning, one might have trouble remembering words, eventually progressing to the point where he has trouble comprehending what is spoken and has difficulty forming complete sentences. It can affect the ability to move, producing slow or jerky movements or loss of balance. The brain's ability to keep bodily systems running smoothly might deteriorate, creating sudden drops in blood pressure, lapses of consciousness, or susceptibility to infections.

The progressive downhill slide means the individual has to continually adjust to greater and greater levels of cognitive deficits. The erosions to learning and reasoning skills diminish one's ability to cope with the increasing decline, leading to the need for more and more help. There is great variability in the exact order of the deficits lost and the steepness of the decline due to our individual uniqueness. The underlying reasons will be addressed in Chapter 3 Dementia's Assault on the Brain.

As I drove Mom's car from her house in New York to our home in Wisconsin, I reflected on the years Mom had taken care of her mother-in-law and her Aunt Anna, who had raised her. Now, it was our turn to take care of her. I remembered an old TV series, *The Walton's*, and their multigenerational family. I was confident this would work for us, or so I thought.

The mom I remembered, the one I thought was coming to live with us, took charge. Her professional career spanned from working as the home economics reporter for a city-wide newspaper to auditing state facilities as a registered dietician. Even in her later years, she fully participated in her church's activities, including helping with vacation Bible school. I had no doubt she would fit right in, network with everyone at church and find her niche in our community.

My mother, as a registered dietician, used to be able to name all the essential amino acids, and list the meatless food combinations that could provide complete proteins in a single meal. She was the great networker, who tracked the comings and goings of our extended family. These abilities melted away before our eyes.

While in many ways she looked and acted just like the mom I remembered, she had changed. Instead of establishing herself in her new community, she stayed home except for excursions to Walgreens. She did not try to make friends at the local senior center or to meet any new people beyond our friends at church. She frequently expressed how she felt left behind. It was as if we lived our lives in the fast lane while she had cruised to a stop on the shoulder of the highway. Some days, it felt like we lived in different time dimensions. I began to wonder if Mom's cognitive difficulties were normal for her age or was something else going on?

I tried to rationalize her difficulties. Didn't everyone lose cognitive abilities with age? But then, I would remember my grandmother had a sharp intellect into her 90s. Was it normal for my mother to struggle with remembering words, organizing her sitting room, or initiating projects?

Although she managed to learn her way around the streets in our small community, we grew increasingly concerned about her safety and well-being while we were at work. She didn't seem to be eating the lunches I left for her. We worried she might slip and fall when taking a shower alone at home. She could no longer send emails without help. While I kept hoping her mental acuity would return once she settled into life in Wisconsin, it seemed to deteriorate as the days went by.

Once we suspect dementia, we need to consider whether it could be *normal brain aging* rather than dementia. Are there signs we can identify that will help point us toward what's going on with our loved ones? What are the warning signs? What are the differences between normal brain aging and dementia? Where does it cross the line into progressive dementia? Let's begin with normal brain aging.

What Does Normal Brain Aging Look Like?

We slow down as we age: we cannot run as fast, our response time slows and we cannot respond to that green light as quickly as we once did, chores take longer and exhaust us more quickly than they used to.

Similar changes occur with our mental acuity or sharpness, as well. It takes longer to recall a fact or to learn new information. We lose our train of thought and have to stop mid-sentence to try to recall what we had intended to say. We can picture a common object in our mind, but have to work to recall its name. We momentarily forget where we are and struggle to remember the purpose for our trip. Where did we park our car in the parking lot this time? We have to concentrate harder and deliberately map out the landmarks around

Normal Brain Aging or Dementia?

our car before we walk into the store. Time seems to fly by as our mental processes slow down. It takes longer to get anything done.

With age, the fluid in our cells decreases. Recent research has demonstrated our brain cells do not die off, but their replacement rate slows and cell size shrinks. At the same time, we produce fewer neurotransmitters (neurons are not connected, but transmit signals using chemical messengers that cross the gaps).[2] It takes longer to reason and to recall information. This decrease in function makes it harder to concentrate and focus. We are more easily distracted.

Normal brain aging will not interfere with our abilities to complete daily tasks, initiate multi-step projects, balance our checkbooks, handle our finances, understand abstract concepts and reasoning, or make sound decisions, though it may take us longer. We do find our car and recognize it when we see it. We can retrace our steps to find our glasses. We remember a forgotten name as we go to sleep that night.

Normal brain aging means we will have to do things differently. We will have to plan more, rely on organizational aids, multitask less (greater difficulty focusing means we have to pay attention as we accomplish a task), and realize everything will take more time. Just as we need more time to clear the weeds out of the back lot or can the bushel of just-picked peaches, we need to allow for the changes in our aging brain. However normal brain aging does not impact our ability to live independently.

Is It Normal Brain Aging or Dementia?

In order to discern whether our loved one has normal brain aging or dementia, we have to analyze his present behaviors with past abilities. If someone was prone to getting lost, becoming confused while negotiating multiple city interchanges might not be a sign of dementia, just poor navigation skills. If he tends to be a little scatterbrained or absent-minded, this might just be a bad day for him, not the beginnings of dementia.

Since in the past, Mom could be somewhat absent-minded, such as making shopping lists and never remembering to take them with her to the store, I initially discounted many of the signs. In addition, the mental decline of someone who is extremely intelligent may decrease her abilities to the level of the average person, making it easy to miss the early signs of dementia (this type of individual usually passes the in-office tests for dementia while in the early stages). No one exhibits all of the warning signs at the beginning.

Cognitive Areas Affected by Dementia

Cognitive areas that might be affected by dementia are:

1. Ability to remember recent events or facts
2. Ability to converse
3. Ability to correctly perceive the world and react to it
4. Ability to plan and complete tasks
5. Ability to initiate actions
6. Ability to make good decisions
7. Ability to use numbers and calculate
8. Ability to reason abstractly
9. Ability to empathize with others
10. Sudden shifts in personality

These cognitive deficits can produce: forgetfulness of recent events; hesitancy to engage in conversation; not recognizing close friends or family; getting lost in familiar places; loss of interest in activities or hobbies; making bad decisions, especially with money; paranoia, delusions, or hallucinations; or callous indifference or thoughtlessness.

1. Ability to Remember Recent Events or Facts

It is normal to temporarily forget names, or not recall some detail when one has not been paying attention. However, not being able to recall recent events is a sign of cognitive impairment. Your loved one might remember going to the store and forget what he did there. He will repeatedly ask the same question since he does not remember asking it or the answer.

Other signs that our loved one is struggling with short-term memory are: frequently losing her train of thought, increased difficulty participating in conversations, increased use of memory aids such as Post-it® Notes and calendars. Since she will not recall recent events or conversations, she might insist you overlooked inviting her to an important family event, or that you talked with her about a certain topic. She might deny saying something you know she said.

When Mom moved in with us we had to transfer her direct deposits to our local bank. Mom and I completed most of the transfers from home except for one that had no online form. The teller at the bank told me that Mom had to go in and request the transfer herself. My working full time made this difficult. Since the bank was easy to find, I thought she could do this herself during the day.

That morning, I gave her detailed written instructions and made sure she had all the documents she needed. I pointed out the route on her map as I highlighted the location of the bank branch.

"OK, Mom, can you get this done today?"

Mom, nodded, smiled, and gave me her usual peck on the cheek as I headed out the door. "Sure thing. See you tonight, Honey."

"Great, Mom," I replied, feeling relieved.

While cooking supper that night, I asked her, "How did it go at the bank?"

"The bank?"

"Did you get your direct deposit transferred?"

"I don't know."

I turned from the fridge, speechless. I did have the presence of mind to close the fridge door and place the casserole on the counter. "OK, did you go to the bank today?"

"I think so. Yes, I went." Mom smiled.

"Great. What did you do there?"

"I don't remember," she said flatly.

A shiver ran down my spine. She could not remember what she had done at the bank. Anything could have happened to her and she would not have known enough to tell us. "Well, OK. How about chicken casserole for supper? Let's get the coffee going."

I made a point of getting off work early enough the next day to run to the bank. Thankfully, she had successfully transferred her direct deposit and all was well, but my nerves were still on edge. What else could she not remember?

2. Ability to Converse

While it's normal to forget a name, we will eventually remember it, even if it happens in the middle of the night. Having difficulty searching for a word or experiencing momentary lapses are the inconvenient reality of aging, but we can still communicate verbally and are not hesitant about joining conversations. As we age, we have to focus more on paying attention. Letting our minds wander can cause us to lose our train of thought. However, with some cues, we will recall enough of the conversation to keep going.

Problems with language, such as having trouble crafting sentences or understanding conversations, are early signs of dementia. Is he quieter than usual and participating less in conversations? Does he struggle to remember common words or use unusual words to name common objects? He might call a "watch" a "hand clock." He also might struggle with remembering what words mean. For example, he won't be able to respond when you ask him to hand you a fork if he has forgotten what the word means.

3. Ability to Correctly Perceive the World and React to It

Even if our brains are slowing down, we can still learn new concepts and update our internal self-image. When we make mistakes, we can self-correct or learn from the input of others to adjust our perceptions. Even if we momentarily lose track of where we are or our destination, utilizing the clues around us, we can reorient ourselves and continue on our journey. If we lose something, we can retrace our steps to find it.

However, with dementia, the parts of the brain that seamlessly match our inner reality to the outside world may become impaired. Depending upon the disease(s) involved, our loved one might not understand she is forgetting things, might not be able to analyze where a missing item might be, or might become confused to where or when she is (called *disorientation to time and place*). She can create stories to explain the world as she sees it—someone is breaking into her house and leaving empty glasses on the countertop—even though they often make no sense. No amount of explaining or reasoning can change her mind.

Disorientation to time erodes understanding of the context of daily events. Your loved one might lose the ability to understand what the time of day or season means. She no longer comprehends that 5 p.m. means it's almost suppertime, or that leaves falling from the trees signify fall is here and winter is approaching.

Disorientation to place can lead to becoming lost in familiar areas. It's normal to get lost in unfamiliar areas, but it is a warning sign when one gets lost on the way to the neighborhood grocery store or bank, or in a relative's house.

Misplacing items repeatedly throughout the day and not being able to retrace one's steps to find them is an early warning sign of dementia. My sister Joan drove up to our parents' retirement home in northern New York state to help Mom while Dad went through his surgery. While there, Dad gave Joan a set of instructions which included how to keep Mom from losing things. She lost her hearing aids multiple times throughout each day and would leave her purse in a store. Dad tried valiantly to teach Mom to always put these items in the same place so she could find them later, but it never worked.

The brain loses track because it has a harder time paying attention, cannot remember recent events and has increasing trouble recalling maps for the location of items. Additionally, she might have been put it in an unusual spot, such as leaving the frying pan in the bathroom.

Another sign is to accuse others of taking lost items. A healthy brain will be able to accept responsibility and reason out a solution.

4. Ability to Plan and Complete Tasks

Getting dressed, making breakfast, placing a telephone call or mowing the lawn seem like simple tasks until you list the cognitive steps required for completion. When the brain no longer remembers one or more of the crucial steps involved, or the order required, tasks cannot be completed.

Remembering how to do things is called *procedural memory*. Some abilities, such as being able to play hymns on a piano may remain while others, such as safely cooking breakfast, may vanish. It's hard to admit dementia's existence when your loved one can sit at the piano and play hymns from memory. However, noticing problems in key areas like being able to pay bills, cook safely or perform routine household maintenance point to the presence of cognitive decline.

Another issue lies with uneven abilities from day to day, or hour to hour. A person showing signs of dementia might be able to function fairly well in the morning, but grow confused in the afternoon. Some days she seems just fine, while on other days she cannot recognize close family and friends. Many people appear quite capable during a brief shopping trip, but might not be able to do anything else except lie on the couch until the next morning. Her fluctuating capabilities can produce family friction as those who see her briefly during her good times might not recognize her cognitive difficulties.

In the past Mom emailed her grandchildren. Knowing she wanted to continue to communicate via email, we set up her computer in her sitting room and made sure the quick link to her email account was on her desktop.

When she had trouble accessing her email, I showed her the

quick link and opened it. She could not remember what to do next, so I showed her the steps for finding her inbox and the button for composing a new email. I assumed all was well.

The next day, she told me she could not do email. I wrote notes for the emailing steps and posted them on her monitor. A few days later, she informed me she couldn't send her emails. The notes had disappeared and I went through the instructions again. I was mystified why my intelligent mother could no longer navigate her email account.

5. Ability to Initiate Activities

Inability to begin activities or respond appropriately is called apathy and can occur early with some diseases causing dementia. Studies have shown that apathy caused by dementia is not related to depression or other psychiatric problems. Persistent apathy, apart from any identifiable causes, might point to dementia.[3] However, other conditions such as dehydration or cardiovascular issues could be responsible.[4] Ask a doctor to investigate the root cause(s) if you see decreases in activity.

My husband and I renovated two bedrooms for my mother's use: one became her bedroom, and the other was her sitting room with her computer, desk, bookcase and a winged-back chair. At first, she found places for things and organized her bedroom fairly well. However, a month later, she found it hard to organize her sitting room. I tried to help by providing a filing box and labeling file drawers, leaving her notes when I went to work. Thinking the number of unpacked boxes crowding her room overwhelmed her, I squirreled most of the boxes away and selected only a few for her to work on each day.

Nothing helped. She spent her days in her sitting room shuffling papers from one pile to another, hoarding paper, cutting them into pieces and piling them around her chair. She seemed to have lost the initiative to unpack and organize. Day by day the room's clutter increased.

6. Ability to Make Good Decisions

What separates a momentary lapse in judgment from a sign of encroaching dementia is awareness of events and the ability to learn from mistakes. Anyone can fall victim to a con artist, but this experience should increase our knowledge of such situations so we will be less likely fooled the next time. We can put remedies in place to improve our future decision-making.

When dementia is involved, she may not even admit the event happened or that it was a mistake. She will not be able to learn from the situation, but will make the same mistakes over and over again. We all vary in our abilities to make "good" decisions. However, a sudden drop in our normal level of decision-making is a sign something is going on with our brains.

Decreasing ability to make good decisions often shows up with mishandling of money or not dressing properly for the weather or occasion. Not recognizing telemarketing scams, forgetting to pay bills or choosing clothes inappropriate for the weather demonstrate decreased ability to make sound decisions. Increasing incidents of poor judgment point to dementia.

7. Ability to Use Numbers and Calculate

We take the cognitive ability required to reference and manipulate numbers for granted. While our ability to do math in our heads or the speed we are able to calculate diminishes, we can still balance the checkbook, solve equations or analyze spreadsheets.

Abstract concepts, including numbers, how to compute them and keep track of dates become harder to grasp with dementia. The numbers in the squares on the calendar might begin to lose their relationship with life. If your loved one is now unable to balance the checkbook or no longer able to use a calendar to plan the day, dementia might be to blame. This can happen even if he was a math whiz in the past.

8. Ability to Reason Abstractly

Abstract thinking involves noticing similarities to form rules or outcomes that can be applied to new or different situations. We use abstract thinking to generalize rules we have learned in the past to solve future problems.

If our loved one is having troubles in abstract reasoning, she will not be able to apply logic to solve problems.

When my sister Ann visited Mom at Sienna Crest, Mom told her they had to go back to Walgreen's to get her keys. Ann was perplexed since she had seen Mom's car in the facility's parking lot when she arrived. Ann tried to prove the keys had to be in Mom's room, but this reasoning was now beyond her. Only when they returned to Walgreen's and the pharmacy technician assured her the keys were not in the store was she willing to search her room where the keys were found.

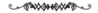

9. Ability to Empathize with Others

Coming alongside someone to encourage them requires analysis of her mood and feelings as expressed by her body language, intonation and word choices. Knowing the context of the situation, our friend's history, combined with other data helps us respond with care and compassion when she is in need.

This ability can be impaired if your loved one no longer perceives the feelings of others by watching their body language. Putting emotion in our language and body gestures can be degraded, as well. While our loved one might intellectually perceive we are struggling with emotional difficulties, she might not be able to respond with empathy. For example, a woman in the early stages might be able to get her husband to the hospital if he is injured in an accident, but will not extend any concern or caring. She might even be puzzled by his display of emotions over a serious injury such as the loss of a finger.

10. Sudden Shifts in Personality

Is it normal to become irritable and short-tempered as we age? Should we expect our basic personalities to change? The Baltimore Longitudinal Study of Aging (BLSA) demonstrated that adult personalities do not change much after 30.[5] While anyone can have a bad day or act out of character compared to his baseline personality, eventually he returns to his normal behavior.

However, a person with dementia can go through rapid and unexplained mood swings ranging from anger to calm to tears within a few moments.[6] He can have catastrophic reactions out of proportion to the situation.[7] This might indicate dementia beginning in the frontal lobes.

Dramatic changes to a person's basic personality points to dementia when he begins displaying unusual behavior such as suspicion, anxiety, obsessiveness, inflexibility, withdrawal or sluggishness. If he does not reset to his baseline personality and these episodes become more frequent, dementia becomes probable.

Another sign of dementia in some individuals is the appearance of social disinhibitions. With some diseases that cause dementia, the control in social situations developed over a lifetime erodes and he begins to act out, seemingly oblivious to the consequences.

Clara looked at Todd, her great-grandson and stated loudly, "He's not normal."

Conversation stopped. Todd's parents froze. Hoping Todd had not heard, the family tried to redirect the conversation, but they were furious. Not recognizing that Clara, the matriarch of the family, was struggling with dementia, the family turned it into an issue. Some of the family members even considered canceling future family gatherings.

Able to Live Independently

Normal brain aging may be embarrassing, reduce a person's efficiency, slow him down, or cause a temporary problem, but it will not disrupt a person's life and ability to live on his own. While he might have to make accommodations for a slower brain and can't quite multi-task the way he used to, he can still manage his own life.

However, with dementia as mental abilities are affected your loved one will find it harder to safely live alone. For example, he might not to remember to take medications in a timely fashion, pay bills, turn off the stove, identify scams, or find his way home. The entrance of progressive cognitive decline means a person's life will necessarily progress to greater dependence on others.

Is Dementia a Possibility?

If your loved one has recently suffered from a serious illness, a fall or a change in life (such as a spouse dying), it might not be dementia. Since normally aging brain cells are smaller and produce fewer neurotransmitters, illnesses, fatigue or grief can bring on transitory problems with cognition. Once he has a chance to heal and adjust, his personality and cognitive abilities should return to normal. Give him time to stabilize—he just might need a little short-term help through a difficult period.

However, if after a period of time he does not recover and his cognitive challenges remain, encourage him to visit a doctor to rule out other causes before settling on a diagnosis such as Alzheimer's. Not everyone with dementia symptoms has a terminal illness. Certain treatable conditions or diseases can also produce these symptoms. If caught in time, the cognitive issues might be resolved. Professional medical advice is critical to taking the necessary steps to find solutions. If the diagnosis does not seem to fit, push for further investigation or seek out other doctors.

The next chapter will describe other causes that can produce dementia symptoms. Knowledge is power and helps us find our way.

Where there is no guidance, a people falls,
but in an abundance of counselors there is safety.
Proverbs 11:14

---

[1] National Institute of Neurological Disorders and Stroke, "Dementia InformationPage." www.ninds.nih.gov/disorders/dementias/dementia.htm. Accessed 9/3/2017.

[2] National Institute on Aging, "How the Aging Brain Affects Thinking." www.nia.nih.gov/health/how-aging-brain-affects-thinking. Accessed 9/3/2017.

[3] H Cerqueira Guimarães, R Levy, A Lúcio Teixeira, R Gomes Beato, and P Caramelli, (2008). "Neurobiology of apathy in Alzheimer's disease." Arquivos de Neuro-Psiquiatria 66(2-B):436-443. http://www.scielo.br/scielo.php?pid=S0004-282X2008000300035&script=sci_arttext. Accessed 9/3/2017.

[4] Peter J Whitehouse, MD, PhD and Daniel George, MSc., *The Myth of Alzheimer's: What You Aren't Being Told about Today's Most Dreaded Diagnosis* (New York: St Martin's Griffin, 2008), pp 186-187.

[5] National Institute on Aging, "Biology of Aging: Research Today for a Healthier Tomorrow," Publication No. 11-7561, November, 2011.

[6] Lela Knox Shanks, *Your Name Is Hughes Hannibal Shanks: A Caregiver's Guide to Alzheimer's* (Lincoln, NE: University of Nebraska Press, 1999), p 17.

[7] Whitehouse and George, p 184.

2

Dementia Basics

After Mom stated she might have Alzheimer's, I told a friend whose mother had been diagnosed with the disease.

When I described my mother's symptoms, she replied, "Oh, she doesn't have Alzheimer's if she's aware she has a problem."

I felt relieved but mystified. Believing that not having Alzheimer's meant she did not have dementia caused me to miss the signs and to expect more from her than what she was capable of handling.

Despite my attempts to help her, Mom's mental functions continued to deteriorate. I took her to see her doctor, hoping for some cure. He administered the Mini-Mental State Exam (MMSE): she knew she was in Wisconsin, but did not remember the name of the town; she remembered the month, but not the day or the year; she could not draw the face of a clock or repeat a list of three items a few minutes later.

Mom's doctor searched for alternative causes, but he did not find any treatable condition for her mental decline. He suggested she try the prescription drug Aricept®, commonly used for treating Alzheimer's.

Mom said, "I already tried that and it made me nervous."

So, someone suspected dementia but never openly discussed it with her before she moved in with us. Instead, she clung to her former doctor's assessment that she did not have Alzheimer's, and tried to overcome her difficulties by making lists and notes and worrying about forgetting.

I went through her long list of medications and eliminated those she no longer needed; but her downward spiral continued. It appeared that Mom had more than just normal brain aging. It felt like a disease had settled into her mind and it seemed like her doctor back in New York had suspected it.

Despite her lack of progress, I kept hoping she would get better. After all, Mom had lost her companion of 50 years, as well as her home and community. Perhaps, in time, she would get past the mourning period and return to her old self, even though it did not appear she had slid into a deep depression. Mom's great faith in God sustained her—she knew her soulmate was in heaven. She was at peace, even though she missed him greatly. Despite how well everything worked out with her move to Wisconsin, her mental capabilities continued to slide.

<hr>

While we can point to reasons or short-term justifications for our loved ones' cognitive difficulties, if the issues do not eventually resolve, it's time to visit the doctor. Dementia symptoms indicate something is going on in the body. Many diseases, aside from Alzheimer's disease, can produce symptoms that look like dementia. Some of them may be treatable. Other mental states, such as delirium or mild cognitive impairment, can resemble dementia.

The next step is to determine if the symptoms could indicate one of the following: delirium; mild cognitive impairment (MCI has few cognitive deficits that do not interfere with daily life); a treatable disease causing dementia-like symptoms ("reversible" dementias); or the probability of dementia.

If your loved one has a treatable condition, the sooner the diagnosis is made and treatment started, the better. Even if the diagnosis is Alzheimer's disease or another similar disease, identifying the cause will point toward the most effective treatments available, as well as give the family time to prepare for the future.

Delirium Might Look Like Dementia

Delirium produces mental confusion that comes and goes suddenly. It is characterized by confusion, disorientation, inability to focus and to maintain consciousness. The symptoms are caused by a passing physiological condition instead of neurological brain damage.

Delirium can occur in the elderly due to normal brain-aging. The changes to their neurons, with fewer neuro-transmitters and synapses, make them susceptible to delirium when the body is under stress.

Delirium, in contrast to dementia, produces altered states of consciousness. People with dementia can usually stay awake and take in stimuli. While they may not interpret their surroundings accurately, they usually do not drift in and out of consciousness. One notable exception occurs with Lewy body dementia that can bring on episodic loss of consciousness.

Stressors such as a urinary tract infection, certain medications, drug interactions, a drop in sodium level, or an electrolyte imbalance in the blood can cause delirium. "Delirium might be the only sign a resident has an infection. Since many elderly do not develop fevers with infections, delirium is often the first sign that something's wrong."[8] Once the underlying cause of the delirium resolves, the mental confusion dissipates and the person regains his normal mind. Delirium comes on suddenly and can leave just as quickly.

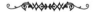

A few days before my father-in-law died of pneumonia, we drove my mother-in-law to the hospital for a visit. As we sat down next to his hospital bed, it shocked us when he accused us of abusing him by taking him to the hospital. When we told him we loved him, he vehemently told us we hated him. The nurse, listening outside in the hall, took us aside and told us he was delirious. The next day, my father-in-law's lucidity returned and he apologized for what he had said the day before. We praised God for a chance to have him back.

Mild Cognitive Impairment (MCI) – Not Quite Dementia

Some people seem to hover between normal brain aging and dementia. With MCI, memory difficulties are usually mild and the loved one can live independently. The mental impairment typically affects a single cognitive ability, such as memory or language. She can still manage her household and her finances, but her cognitive difficulties go beyond normal aging. [9]

At present, doctors cannot tell if MCI will eventually develop into dementia. [10] They cannot predict which individuals will recover to previous levels, stay the same, or continue on to dementia.

"Reversible" Dementias

"Reversible" dementia usually refers to those diseases which produce dementia-like symptoms typically not caused by damage to the brain. The underlying disease or condition produces the dementia symptoms as a secondary cause. Treat the root cause and, often, you can reverse or mitigate the dementia if you catch it in time. However, even with treatment, some people eventually go on to develop dementia in the future.

Treatable conditions with dementia symptoms are: normal pressure hydrocephalus; internal imbalances such as of the thyroid or electrolytes; low vitamin B-12 levels; side effects of prescription drugs or interactions; and problems arising from diabetes, the kidneys, or inadequate nutrition or hydration. [11] Problems in other areas of our bodies can affect our ability to think and reason. Since many other diseases can generate cognitive difficulties, request the doctor to rule out possible treatable conditions with a complete history, office visit, and laboratory tests.[12]

However, some people eventually develop dementia even after treatment. They will see some improvement, but may eventually experience increasing cognitive difficulties. Even if the dementia is not fully reversible, any improvement in symptoms providing more time is of value. This section discusses the most common conditions that can produce reversible dementia.

Deficiencies

Deficiencies and imbalances can create memory problems. Vitamin B-12 is the most common vitamin deficiency. Once identified by a blood test and treated, mental acuity can return to normal.

Other chemical imbalances, such as low or high thyroid levels, can also be discovered through blood tests and treated.

Polypharmacy—Drug Sensitivities or Interactions

Many elderly people have multiple health conditions, and may take several prescription drugs and supplements. Some of the most commonly prescribed prescription drugs can cause confusion. Sometimes, doctors fail to take the physiology of their elderly patients into account and prescribe a larger dose than their kidneys or circulatory system can handle.[13] Drugs and supplements build up in the body and can interact with one another.

Discuss prescription drugs and supplements with the doctor to find any that can be eliminated; some drugs might not be necessary at this stage of life or perhaps the dosages should be adjusted.

When my father-in-law began experiencing increasing cognitive difficulties, his wife carefully went through all the prescriptions he was taking. Sure enough, a number of them caused confusion. Working with his doctors, his wife eliminated the suspect drugs or reduced the dosage. His mental acuity returned. It was good to play card games with them again—one of their favorite social activities.

Normal Pressure Hydrocephalus (NPH)

With NPH, fluid accumulates in the brain, increasing the ventricles (cavities) in the brain and squeezing the brain's cells. This can produce symptoms such as difficulty thinking, processing information, and paying attention, along with impaired walking and balance, which may be confused with Parkinson's disease. However, when given enough time, the person with NPH can still respond to questions.[14]

Mental abilities should improve and the dementia resolve with the installation of a shunt for the excess cerebral spinal fluid (current method of treatment). The degree of recovery varies, depending upon the existence of underlying dementia. In some individuals additional cognitive difficulties can arise in the future. [15]

Depression

Depression slows the brain, makes it difficult to think, and produces a mental fog. Some of the symptoms of depression are similar to the signs of dementia: having difficulty concentrating; experiencing fatigue and decreased energy; showing irritability, restlessness, and loss of interest in activities.[16]

These symptoms can be mistaken for signs of dementia. Since depression often accompanies dementia in the beginning, an in-office test for cognitive issues may identify those individuals with depression only. The cognitive abilities of those without dementia should improve with treatment for depression. While it is common for those with depression to worry if they have dementia, this is rarer for those with dementia.

While, statistically, depression is a risk factor for dementia, studies have not been able to demonstrate that depression causes dementia, or dementia causes depression. However, depression can be an early sign of dementia. After treatment for depression, some people saw cognitive improvements but eventually developed dementia.[17] More recent studies discovered that as dementia symptoms increased, people became less depressed as their abilities to perceive the context of experience waned.[18]

Diseases that Cause Dementia

So, despite our hopes and prayers, the doctors do not find a treatable condition that a shot of vitamin B-12, medications, or a medical procedure can solve. Our loved one's cognitive deficits reach beyond mild cognitive impairment to affecting her daily life.

Presently, no tests exist that definitively diagnose progressive dementia. The doctors make diagnosis of the disease(s) causing the dementia by ruling out other causes. If you question a diagnosis for your loved one and your doctor will not look for treatable causes, it's advisable to obtain a second opinion.

If doctors rule out other causes, there is still a benefit in a diagnosis, even though presently no cures exist. A diagnosis helps the family understand the loved one's puzzling or disturbing behaviors, and they can begin to find treatments to minimize the symptoms. The different diseases which cause dementia progress at varying rates, affect different areas of the brain, and react differently to drugs and therapies. If your loved one's dementia can be diagnosed early enough, your family will have time to plan ahead while your loved one can still express her preferences.

Identifying which disease(s) are causing dementia is a matter of studying people's cognitive difficulties. Your loved one's abilities and behaviors will point to the areas of the brain affected, revealing the most likely disease(s) involved. Since there are few imaging tests that can differentiate among the various dementias, categorizing the behavioral deficits and their order of appearance provides clues to the disease(s) involved (researchers are working on developing imaging tests that can screen for particular diseases).

Two simple in-office mental status tests are commonly used to detect cognitive issues: the *Mini-Mental State Examination* (MMSE) and the *Montreal Cognitive Assessment* (MoCA). The doctor may ask a series of questions to determine several things: if she knows where and when she is, if she can describe her symptoms, if she can remember a short list of objects after a brief period of time, count and manipulate numbers, and draw a clock face. These simplified exams can be performed in most doctors' offices.

Many people with early dementia and MCI may hide or be unaware of the extent of their deficits. The MMSE measures the level of cognitive impairment and can track the decline over a period of time, but it cannot identify the type of dementia and sometimes misses dementia in the early stages. The MoCA, similar to the MMSE, has been more effective in identifying MCI and dementias in the mild, beginning stages.[19]

The most common diseases causing dementia are *Alzheimer's disease, vascular cognitive impairment, Lewy body dementia,* and *frontotemporal dementia.* These are broad categories for several diseases. Other neurodegenerative diseases, such as Parkinson's and Huntington's, may eventually produce dementia symptoms in later stages, but not always. These diseases are terminal and often take years to run their course—sometimes as long as 20 years or more.

The devil's in the details and there are not many for doctors to rely on. Adding to the difficulty is the reality that many people with dementia have two or more diseases operating simultaneously. For example, someone may exhibit symptoms for both vascular cognitive impairment and Alzheimer's disease. Initially, someone with Lewy body or frontotemporal dementia can be misdiagnosed with depression, Parkinson's, or psychosis until doctors discover the actual culprit. The wide range of symptoms can make it hard to exactly determine the diseases present.[20]

Alzheimer's Disease (AD)

With AD, cognitive deficits due to loss of cells in the brain develop so gradually that we recognize them only in hindsight. Unlike other dementias, which can arise suddenly and progress more rapidly, AD sneaks up on a family. No one can pinpoint when the troubles start. Decline becomes evident only by comparing their loved one's current and past abilities.

Carol is a friend of mine whose mother had Alzheimer's disease. She recalled a time when she was on a business trip to Hawaii. She dutifully called her mother each night to ask what she ate for supper and made sure everything was okay, since they lived together.

Her mother, Mary, never sounded upset or asked where she was. After all, Carol had told her mom she was in Hawaii on a business trip. When she returned to her desk at work, she was surprised to find twenty-eight voicemails from her mother asking what to have for supper, but she never asked where her daughter was or why she had not come home.

As Carol thought about what this might mean, she recalled her mother never became upset and still appeared able to function with her daily life.

Deep down she knew something was wrong. "I knew she was having problems at that time. I hid money in my drawer at home so she would have cash if she needed it." Looking back, she began to perceive her mother might have dementia. This was two years before Mary was officially diagnosed with Alzheimer's disease.

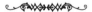

Although AD usually begins with loss of recent memory and progressing to problems performing multistep tasks, reasoning, and personality changes, the exact expression of Alzheimer's can vary greatly from person to person and run its course from two to twenty years.[21] Your loved one may repeat herself, might forget what her closest relatives or friends look like, become lost in familiar areas, have trouble completing tasks, misplace things, or begin to withdraw from social interaction. Some people develop paranoia and become aggressive while others grow sweet and congenial.

Dr. Barry Reisberg of New York University developed a seven-stage model of Alzheimer's progression. While studying the behavioral development of patients, he discovered the typical Alzheimer's progression occurred in the reverse order of development from infancy to adulthood, calling it *retrogenesis*.[22] His seven-stage model has become the standard for determining the functional level of a person with Alzheimer's. However, few patients follow the pattern exactly. Most experience their own unique mix of disease symptoms and progression.

Following Dr. Reisberg's progression, it usually starts with increasing forgetfulness and concentration difficulties. As mental abilities decline, it becomes harder to reason, find solutions to problems, remember directions and locations, and recall facts and events. It becomes harder to complete everyday tasks such as dressing, cooking a meal, or going to the bathroom. Total care is required at the end of life.[23]

Most are diagnosed with Alzheimer's disease after age 65 and more often in women than men. When it occurs before the age of 65, it is called early onset Alzheimer's.[24] It is usually a slow disease with steady decline over the years. Some with early onset might have a shorter progression of five years or so.

Vascular Cognitive Impairment (VCI)

Vascular cognitive impairment (VCI), also known as vascular dementia, is caused by interrupted or degraded blood flow to the brain from a blood clot, or ruptured or leaking arteries.[25] Unlike strokes that affect particular regions of the brain, VCI develops from degeneration in broad regions and produces difficulties in multiple areas that can appear to come and go.

For example, my mother had trouble recalling words, had sporadic short-term memory loss (I could never predict what she would or would not remember), along with periodic inability to analyze situations or make decisions. Her cognitive abilities fluctuated with episodes of sudden decrease in function, leading to being bed-bound for days at a time, only to rebound, but never fully recovering. With VCI, the family can recall when the loss of function occurred, followed by a period of gradual improvement. However, abilities do not return to the level seen before the event.[26] VCI produces episodes of sharp decline with some recovery of abilities. This cycle repeats itself as mental abilities erode until the loved one becomes totally incapacitated.

The symptoms depend upon which areas of the brain are affected. It often occurs in conjunction with other diseases, such as AD, or Lewy body dementia. My mother had symptoms for both AD and VCI.

Mom went through episodes where she could hardly get out of bed. I would call my sisters, thinking she was approaching the end, but by the time they visited, she had bounced back. While she lost ground, she regained some of her abilities.

One time, I apologized to my sister Joan for calling, but she told me I gave her a good excuse to visit and they had a great time.

It felt like I was living on a roller coaster. Is this the end? No, not yet, but I wondered what the future held and how long she would linger.

We took precautions to reduce strokes, since this was a risk factor. She had a prescription to control her blood pressure and her blood work tested in the normal range. Her recurring mini-episodes pointed to silent mini-strokes. Not all VCI can be eliminated.

Frontotemporal Dementia (FTD)

Frontotemporal dementia refers to a cluster of diseases affecting the frontal or temporal lobes (areas in the front or the sides of the head). Where the dementia begins, such as in the frontal lobes, left temporal or right temporal, indicates which disease is involved. The location is determined by the set of behavioral symptoms that develop.[27] The memory areas are usually not affected until later. It can occur as early as forty years old, and is more likely to occur in men than in women.[28]

This disease begins either with behavior, movement, or speech problems, depending upon the lobe that is affected first. Your loved one might begin behaving erratically and appear out of character to his previous personality, develop repetitive behaviors, have difficulty moving, speaking, or understanding what you are saying.[29] Speech difficulties may include not being able to find the right words, incorrect use of grammar resulting in nonsensical speech, or not being able to comprehend what they hear.

Sometimes, their personalities reverse. A sociable person can become introverted; or a modest person may begin exhibiting inappropriate behavior, such as crude, insensitive, or suggestive remarks; demonstrate lack of respect for policemen or employers; or begin stealing.[30]

This disease fits the three-stage model of early, middle and late. It commonly begins with slow, gradual change in the early stages, with the progression accelerating through the middle and late stages. Eventually, all daily activities are affected, resulting in total dependence.[31]

Lewy Body Dementia (LBD)

With LBD, proteins, called Lewy bodies, form clumps in brain cells. These misfolded proteins interfere with the cells' ability to function. Doctors identify the particular type of LBD by studying the symptoms, indicating the location of the Lewy bodies in the brain.

When Lewy bodies form in the cortex, the outer structures of the brain, and the center of the brain, they cause dementia.[32] This disease is closely related to Parkinson's disease, which is caused by Lewy bodies in the brain stem. People with LBD can have Lewy bodies in the cortex, with dementia symptoms, as well as in the brain stem, with Parkinsonian movement issues.

The dementia symptoms, timing, and disease progression with LBD varies greatly. Physically acting out dreams (rapid eye movement—REM behavior disorder—RBD) is often one of the earliest signs of LBD.[33] The cognitive symptoms include problems focusing attention, difficulty planning and making decisions, confusion, not recognizing family members or friends, along with fluctuating levels of attention and alertness.[34] People with LBD have difficulty retrieving their memories (but can often retain recent memories).[35]

The hallucinations that occur with LBD—sensing events or things that do not exist—are usually visual, but they can also be false sounds or smells. LBD can also impair the body's ability to control basic functions such as blood pressure and heart rate, leading to incontinence, fainting, falls, and constipation. It can cause a masklike face, a slow shuffling walk, tremors, and stiff muscles.[36]

The standard Alzheimer's-type seven-stage model does not fit LBD progression. Your loved one with LBD can go suddenly from interacting well in the doctor's office to being unable to speak, move, or get out of bed for the next day or so. The swift changes resemble a roller coaster ride—can he function or will he be bedridden for a while? He can swing from lucid periods to middle-stage confusion to late-stage deficits all within a day, only to bounce back to early stage capabilities. The three-stage model of early, middle, and late fits better with increasing periods of incapacity until total disability occurs. The hallmark of LBD is pronounced up-and-down swings with overall decline.[37]

LBD can occur as early as age fifty or fifty-five, is more prevalent in men than in women, and is often misdiagnosed as AD.[38] It is important to recognize the existence of LBD, since many people with these diseases do not do well with certain drugs, apart from some typical AD medications. Your loved one can become more sensitive to common medications, or develop catastrophic reactions or Parkinson-type symptoms such as rigidity, immobility, inability to communicate, or even death. Interestingly, some people with LBD often react well to common Alzheimer's drugs.[39]

Mixed Dementia

Mixed dementia refers to people with dementia symptoms from more than one disease type. For example, a loved one with Alzheimer's-type dementia could also have symptoms for LBD.[40] Vascular cognitive impairment (VCI) often develops alongside Alzheimer's disease. When these diseases occur together, it seems to increase the severity and accelerate the progression.[41] While the symptoms for VCI overlap those of AD, the symptoms will vary greatly and may not follow the classic AD progression. My mother had Alzheimer's-type downward progression between her sudden declines from VCI.

Hallmarks for the Four Main Diseases:

Alzheimer's Disease (AD)

- Slow, steady loss of mental abilities, beginning with memory
- Usually begins after sixty-five; more common in women.

Vascular Cognitive Impairment (VCI)

- Sudden steep drops in mental abilities with varying symptoms
- Usually begins between sixty-five and seventy-five; more common in men

Frontotemporal Dementia (FTD)

- Begins with behavioral changes and decision-making difficulties or troubles with speech

- Can begin as early as forty; more common in men

Lewy Body Dementia (LBD)

- Can begin with sleep disorder, hallucinations, reasoning or movement difficulties, with sudden losses of consciousness
- Can begin as early as fifty; more common in men

Before we plunge into ways to cope with dementia's progression, we will explore the brain and memory more fully in Chapter 3: Dementia's Assault on the Brain. Understanding how the diseases shape and change the brain, hindering memories and the recall process, impacting behavior, leading to altered abilities and personalities, helps us empathize with our loved ones. Knowledge of common disease progressions can point to solutions for our loved one's current level and anticipate deficits to come.

However, if you feel ready, skip to Part 2: The Dementia Journey, Chapters 4 through 7, where we will look at the stages of dementia, their characteristics, solutions, and coping mechanisms. Dementia stands apart since it appears to touch the soul and change how our loved ones interact with the world. But, we do not walk alone.

"I will never leave you nor forsake you." Hebrews 13:5

---

[8] Jan Zimmerman, RN, Nursing Administrator, Heritage Homes, Watertown, WI. Interview 5/20/2014.

[9] Ronald Petersen, MD, PhD, *Mayo Clinic Guide to Alzheimer's Disease* (Rochester, MN: Mayo Clinic, 2006), p 173.

[10] Ibid., p 174.

[11] M Tripathi and D Vibha (2009). "Reversible dementias." *Indian Journal of Psychiatry* 51(Suppl1):S52-S55. ww.ncbi.nlm.nih.gov/pmc/articles/ PMC3038529. Accessed 12/1/2016.

12   P Ioannidis and D Karacostas, "How Reversible are 'Reversible Dementias'?" *European Neurological Review*, 2011:6:(4)230-3. www.touchneurology.com/articles/how-reversible-are-reversible-dementias. Accessed 9/4/2017.

13   PA Routledge, MS O'Mahony, and KW Woodhouse (2004). "Adverse drug reactions in elderly patients." *British Journal of Clinical Pharmacology* 57(2):121-126. www.ncbi.nlm.nih.gov/pmc/articles/PMC1884428/. Accessed 5/19/2014.

14   Petersen, p 155.

15   Ibid., p 156.

16   The National Institute of Mental Health, "Depression." www.nimh.nih.gov/health/ topics/depression/index.shtml. Accessed 1/10/2017.

17   Ioannidis and Karacostas.

18   Dennis Thompson, "Light Shed on Link Between Depression, Dementia," www.webmd.com/depression/news/20140730/scientists-shed-light-on-link-between-depression-dementia. Accessed 10/6/2015. Quote from Robert S Wilson citing his study: RS Wilson, AW Capuano, PA Boyle, GM Hoganson, LP Hizel, RC Shah, S Nag, JA Schneider, SE Arnold, and DA Bennett (2014). "Clinical-pathological study of depressive symptoms and cognitive decline in old age." *Neurology* 2014 Aug 19;83(8):702-709. Published online July 30, 2014.

19   PT Trzepacz, H Hockstettler, S Wang, B Walker, AJ Saykin (2015). "Relationship between the Montreal Cognitive Assessment and Mini-mental State Examination for assessment of mild cognitive impairment in older adults," *BMC Geriatrics*. (2015)15:107. www.ncbi.nlm.nih.gov/pubmed/26346644. Accessed 9/4/2017.

20   Petersen, p 51.

21   Ibid., p 65.

22   B Reisberg, EH Franssen, LE Souren, SR Auer, I Akram, and S Kenowsky (2002). "Evidence and mechanisms of retrogenesis in Alzheimer's and other dementias: management and treatment import." *American Journal of Alzheimers Diseases and Other Dementias* 17(4):202-212. www.ncbi.nlm.nih.gov/pubmed/12184509. Accessed 2/3/2017.

23   Dementia Care Central, "Seven Stages of Dementia: Symptoms & Progression." www.dementiacarecentral.com/aboutdementia/facts/stages/. Accessed 2/3/2017.

24   Alzheimer's Association, "What Is Alzheimer's?" www.alz.org/alzheimers_disease_what_is_alzheimers.asp. Accessed 9/4/2017.

25   Petersen, pp 141-142.

26   Tam Cummings, PhD, *Untangling Alzheimer's: The Guide for Families and Professionals (A Conversation in Caregiving)*, 2nd ed., (North Charleston, SC: The Dementia Association LLC, 2015), p 220.

27   The Association for Frontotemporal Degeneration, "The FTD Disorders." www.theaftd.org/understandingftd/disorders. Accessed 1/10/2017.

28   Martin Rossor, MD FRCP, FMedSci, "Chapter 1. The ABCs of Neurodegenerative Dementias," in Gary Radin and Lisa Radin (eds.), *What If It's Not Alzheimer's?:A Caregiver's Guide to Dementia*, 3*rd* ed. (Amherst, NY: Prometheus Books, 2014), p 39.

29   The Association for Frontotemporal Degeneration, "Disease Overview." www.theaftd.org/understandingftd/ftd-overview. Accessed 12/1/2016.

30   The Association for Frontotemporal Degeneration, "Behavioral Variant FTD(bvFTD)." www.theaftd.org/understandingftd/disorders/bv-ftd. Accessed 12/1/2016.

31   Murray Grossman, MD, EdD, " Chapter 2, "What Is Frontotemporal Degeneration?: A Clinical Perspective," in Gary Radin and Lisa Radin (eds.), *What If It's Not Alzheimer's?:A Caregiver's Guide to Dementia*, 3*rd* ed. (Amherst, NY: Prometheus Books, 2014), pp 48-49.

32   National Institutes of Health, "What Is Lewy Body Dementia?" https://www. nia. nih.gov/health/what/lewy-body-dementia. Accessed 9/4/2017.

33   Lewy Body Dementia Association, "Symptoms." ww.lbda.org/content/ symptoms. Accessed 11/30/2016.

34   Petersen, p 131.

35   Helen Buell Whitworth and James Whitworth, *A Caregiver's Guide to Lewy Body Dementia*, (New York: demosHealth, 2011), pp 35-36.

36   Lewy Body Dementia Association, "Symptoms."

37   MedicineNet.com, "Lewy Body Dementia Symptoms and Prognosis." www. medicinenet.com/lewy_body_dementia_lbd_symptoms_and_prognosis/ views/htm. Accessed 9/4/2017.

38   National Institutes of Health, "What Is Lewy Body Dementia?"

39   Lewy Body Dementia Association, "Recent Studies Demonstrate Benefits of Cholinesterase Inhibitors in DLB." https://www.lbda.org/content/ recent-studies-demonstrate-benefits-cholinesterase-inhibitors-dlb. Accessed 9/4/2017. And Whitworth and Whitworth, pp 95-96.

40   Alzheimer's Association, "Mixed Dementia," www.alz.org/dementia/mixed-dementia-symptoms.asp. Accessed 9/4/2017.

41   Petersen, p 145.

3

Dementia's Assault on the Brain

At the beginning of a road trip to her brother's house, my friend Carol was taken aback when her mother said, "I don't know who you are, but you're driving my daughter's car."

Even though she told her mother that she was her daughter, Mary quizzed her repeatedly. "What's your father's name? Where did you go to school? I don't know who you are. What's your brother's name? Do you have a dog?"

She realized the trip might not be a good idea and she feared that she would not be able to get her mother into the car the next morning. So, Carol turned around to go back home.

During that time, Mary continually quizzed Carol, never realizing she was talking to her daughter.

Carol said, "All the way home, she quizzed me about things she thought her daughter would know and she still didn't get it. That's the first time I realized that she did not recognize me. We're talking a period of two hours up the road and two hours down the road."

Dementia leaves a trail of confusion in its wake. Someone with dementia may look and sound so healthy; seem so fit. We remember how our mother, wife, or daughter had been with us and what we meant to her. Then, she begins to speak or act in foreign, unfamiliar ways. It almost seems as if an alien has taken up residence in her body, but we know she's still there.

Our Marvelous Brain

The brain is the junction where our soul and spirit interacts with this world. We use our brains to feel, think, reason, and remember. With our minds, we control our bodies so we can sing, dance, draw, or accomplish a myriad of tasks. The state of our brain affects our ability to function in this physical world. While many systems in the body can work for a while without input from the brain, ultimately, a body cannot maintain life without a brain. It keeps the lungs breathing, and our organs working in unison, making it possible to get up, go to work, fix the car, play with the kids, cook a meal, or walk the dog without concerning ourselves with keeping our bodies alive.

Stimuli from our senses tell us about the physical world around us, and internal sensors tell us how our bodies are doing. We engage in abstract reasoning and can imagine what does not exist. With our mind's eye, we paint a tropical sunset, create heavenly music or foot-tapping rhythms, and reason out a geometry problem. On the conscious level, we plan, remember, and think. Underneath, the subconscious brain runs subroutines that control bodily functions, analyzes ideas, imbeds memories, and solves problems. We hardly notice everything it's doing until parts of the brain begin to weaken and fail.

As a physical organ, our brain will affect how well we can react, move, think, and reason. It's a dance between our choices affecting our brains and our brains affecting our life choices. When the brain begins to fail, eventually it will cause our bodies to fail.

I entered Mom's room at Sienna Crest a week after Thanksgiving and set up her Christmas decorations: her one-piece nativity scene, a musical snow globe, a miniature Christmas tree, and a trio of lighted ceramic angels. Once everything was in place and the angels glowed softly, I set about finding her. This day, she sat in the back living room. Even though a movie was playing, I managed to get her to go to her room, anticipating her delight with her room's transformation.

She said nothing as I led her to her recliner. "Look, it's Christmas," I said, handing her the blue lit angel.

"Oh, that's nice," she stated flatly.

The previous Christmas, she had insisted I give her this set of angels that lit up red, green, and blue. She used to love Christmas and enjoyed seeing her room decked out for the season.

Disappointed and discouraged, I contrasted her present behavior with her excitement about past holidays. I made small talk, but I despaired as I sat with her until it was time to help her to the dining room.

What was the good of all her Bible knowledge and memorized verses if she forgot it all? She didn't even care she no longer went to church with us. The wooden cross on her wall that we had diligently shopped for no longer reminded her of her faith in Christ. I looked again at that simple cross, trying not to dwell on what she had lost. At that time, I did not truly understand she had forgotten God's name, along with the holidays that celebrated His life.

Despite her firmly held beliefs and love of Christ, her failing cognitive abilities, including memory loss and apathy, rendered Christmas too abstract to grasp. Her emotional connection to the decorations seemed to have disappeared, just as she no longer reacted to holding her great-grandson.

I knew she still loved God, even if she forgot His name and the celebration of His birth. "Jesus loves you," I told her repeatedly. It was enough for her. It had to be enough for me. Deep in my soul, I knew God would never leave her, not even in her loss of knowing.

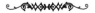

The Cells That Make Up the Brain

The brain, composed of billions of *neuronal* and *glial* cells, is a complex computing device more complicated than the most advanced computer.

Signals from other neurons flow from the dendrites to the neuron's body and out its axon. Most neurons have one axon for transmitting a signal, but several dendrites for reception. If signals need to travel in both directions, neurons from both ends have to lay down axons to carry the signals.

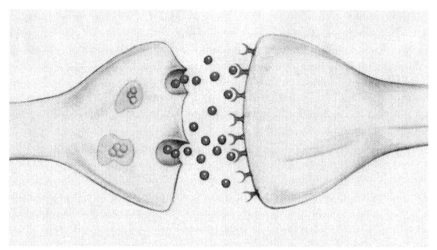

Figure 1 Neurotransmitters jump the gap between axon to dendrite. Illustration by Lindsay J. Billington.

Neurons do not touch each other, but are separated by short gaps between the dendrites and axons called *synapses*. Synaptic ends release *neurotransmitters* to cross the gap.

The other cells in the brain are the glial cells, once considered as simply support cells for the neurons, providing nourishment and structure for the brain's cellular matrix.[42] Until recently, little was known about the glia cell's role in cognition. Recent discoveries revealed the neurons and glia work together in thought and reasoning. The glia cleans out the synaptic gap so another signal can be transmitted, and provides the nutrients the neurons needs.

Glial cells communicate through their calcium channel waves and stimulate the neurons to fire or turn them down.[43]

While the brain has many different types of cells, the best-known types of glial cells are: *astrocytes, oligodendrocytes,* and *microglia.* Astrocytes are the main support cells, creating the connective matrix securing surrounding neurons and axon. They provide nutrients to neurons, remove debris, and respond to brain injury by healing neurons and stimulating synaptic growth. Some astrocytes, still in an undeveloped stage, can transform into neurons or glial cells as needed. Oligodendrocytes wrap the axons in the brain with myelin. One oligodendrocyte will encase many axons with myelin, like many hands with long arms holding onto a group of children. The microglial are the brain's immune cells engulfing microbes and releasing toxins to destroy invaders. They purge unwanted synapses or neurons when rewiring circuits for learning, and provide healing proteins when neurons are injured.[44]

The brain is composed of grey and white matter. The grey matter, in the outer layer, houses most of the cell bodies while the white matter is composed of myelin-coated axonal tracts linking sections together. The outer layer, called the *cerebral cortex,* is organized in horizontal layers of cells arranged in vertical columns. Axons branch out, connecting an area internally, as well as with other areas, near and far.[45]

The Center of the Brain

Information streams into the brain through its center via the brain stem at the top of the spinal column. In the brainstem and the brain's center, signals from throughout the body are processed, analyzed, and routed to corresponding brain areas. The *thalamus,* a key routing hub, is also a relay station for white matter highways, linking different areas within the brain.[46]

The *hypothalamus,* just underneath the thalamus, maintains automatic bodily systems, such as the cardiovascular and digestive systems. For example, the hypothalamus sets the heart rate, blood pressure, blood sugar levels, and indicates when to start and stop eating. This area also houses an internal clock that sets our daily, circadian rhythm, helping us stay awake during the day and become sleepy at night.[47]

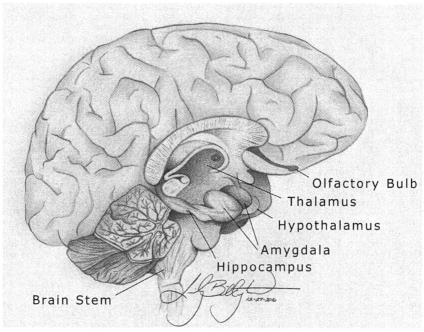

Figure 2 The limbic cortex. Illustration by Lindsay J. Billington.

In the center of the brain, the limbic cortex wraps around the top of the brain stem. This region includes the *hippocampus* and *amygdala*, which are closely tied to the thalamus. Information streams into the hippocampal area where it selects data to index for later memory retrieval as the nearby amygdala assesses threats and danger. The locations of the linked memories are stored in the hippocampus so the event can be retrieved. Sights, sounds, aromas, as well as the feelings experienced during an event are indexed to be remembered later.[48] This structure identifies and updates relevant information.[49]

The hippocampus, in conjunction with the parietal lobe at the top of the brain, tells us where our bodies are in relation to space. Parts of the hippocampus remember where we have been and its location.[50] We utilize these maps to remember where the bathroom is, how to get to the store, and to help us select the best route to a destination. Even getting up from a chair and walking to the kitchen requires selecting the proper internal map.

The hippocampus creates episodic memory—remembering where and when events happened. It can record position and distance traveled or elapsed time, depending upon which factor is more important.[51] This, coupled with the other areas of the brain that track time, helps us to know where and when we are.

The amygdala links emotional experience with the corresponding sensory inputs, identifying fears and dangers. It also helps us identify anger or fear in others.[52] This structure works in a network with the prefrontal cortex, in the front of the frontal lobe, to enable a person to identify threats while controlling responses in conformity with socially acceptable behavior.[53]

The *olfactory bulb* identifies scents and transmits them to the inner surface of the temporal lobe where pertinent data is forwarded on to the hippocampus and amygdala. This creates the strong ties between smell, emotion and memory.[54]

Cerebral Lobes

The cerebrum, which is composed of gray and white matter, envelops the central limbic area as two halves connected by a white matter highway flowing through its center.[55] While the two halves of the brain appear to be mirror images of each other, the left side processes detailed data, logic, and analytical thinking while the right side tends to be more creative, focusing on the whole rather than parts, and embedding feeling and emotion into speech and actions.[56]

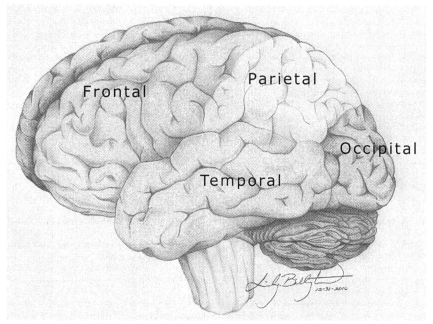

Figure 3 Cerebral lobes. Illustration by Lindsay J. Billington.

Each half is divided into four lobes following the deep grooves in the folded cerebral cortex. The four lobes are: *frontal, temporal, parietal,* and *occipital.*

Through studies of people with brain trauma, scientists have mapped the main jobs or functions of the lobes:[57]

- *Frontal Lobes* (in the front, over the eyes) seem to be the main center for personality, thinking, reasoning, decision-making, emotional control, and movement;
- *Temporal Lobes* (on the sides, above the ears) specialize in memory and tasks related to hearing, speech, and language;
- *Parietal Lobes* (at the top of the brain) process sensory information in relation to physical location, pain, taste, and touch, and is instrumental in planning and executing complex movements; and
- *Occipital Lobes* (in the back of the brain) house the visual cortex for processing visual data.[58]

In parts of the frontal lobes, working memory assembles facts and data with images from the visual cortex, along with principles to develop solutions for problem-solving.[59] The frontal lobes also contain the circuits for movement, initiating action, and in conjunction with the cerebellum, select the proper muscle sequences for the intended action.[60]

The frontal lobes, in conjunction with the parietal and temporal lobes are instrumental for developing our personality. We learn to interpret and anticipate other's emotions and actions. This includes choosing not to react as we would like for the benefit of others. Making conscious choices to control our emotions, we delay our own wants and desires to achieve future goals. We learn how to control our responses, engage in social interactions, develop ways to complete tasks, and initiate plans in key association areas in the frontal lobes, working with other connected areas in the temporal and parietal lobes.

The temporal lobes process incoming sounds, interpret what we hear and create the responses. These areas analyze aromas, as well as certain memory functions.[61] The auditory cortex in the temporal lobes, along with other related areas, sorts through incoming sounds and focuses attention on the target conversation or set of sounds.[62] While the left, analytical side deals with the mechanics of speech, assigning words to objects and creating language, the right side adds emotional content to what we say and helps us interpret underlying emotions.[63]

Sense perception and controlling movement in response to sensory input reside in the parietal lobes and top of the frontal lobes, helping us move through space.[64] They identify the locations of our aches, pain, itches, and tell us if we are hot or cold.[65]

Brain Networks

But, the parts of the brain do not work in isolation. White matter tracts throughout the brain provide the data highways by which information streams in coordinated networks to accomplish tasks. Long-distance axons bundled together into dedicated white matter highways connect key areas throughout the brain for analyzing, processing, and manipulating incoming data. Many networks have been identified, such as those integrating our visual world, speech and sound, working memory, emotion, motor control, and time perception. For example, driving to a destination requires coordination of images from the visual cortex, along with map retrieval from the hippocampus, with instant recall of planned sequences to respond appropriately to the surrounding traffic.

Like a symphony orchestra creating beautiful music from the coordination of many different types of instruments, cognition arises from the interconnections of brain regions. Association areas within a cerebral hemisphere, such as the visual cortex, work together with distant areas in broad networks. Cognition is a result of the networking of far-flung areas of the brain.[66] These master networks oversee activity between the various association areas of the brain.

Many researchers have labeled the main higher level core networks as:

Default mode network (DMN)
Salience network (SN)
Central executive network (CEN).[67]

The default mode network (DMN) includes those areas of brain that are activated when we are not focusing our attention to plan or solve a problem. With this network, we maintain our internal self-image, monitor, and process social responses.[68] We reflect on our memories, reviewing our history in context with the world around us. We are able to take in our current reality, fit it into our past, and anticipate or develop our reactions to the world around us. We know where we are, what we have done today, and what we intend to do. This is where we are when we're enjoying the sunset or doing routine tasks that require little thinking, such as buttoning a shirt.

The salience network (SN) constantly monitors input from our internal and external worlds, looking for important data or situations that require attention and priority. It dynamically switches between the DMN and central executive network (CEN). The CEN runs the show when our attention is focused on problem-solving or thinking.[69]

For example, while walking down the sidewalk on our way to work, the DMN allows our mind to wander, thinking about plans for the weekend or musing about a project, while our unconscious mind oversees routines that monitor the grade, pitch, and firmness of the concrete, adjusting the firing of muscle fibers, ever aware of the internal gyroscope in the inner ear to maintain balance. Simultaneously, other automatic networks regulate blood pressure, glucose levels, heartbeat, and respiration.

The SN, remembering an early meeting coupled with noting the time on the large clock in the main square, shuts down the DMN to activate the CEN. Various routines in the brain compare the estimated time of your arrival at work with the time for the first meeting of the day. To solve the problem of getting to work in time to make the meeting with all your required notes and files, the CEN, utilizing physiological data, maps, and related time sequencing, devises a plan and sets it in motion. The SN dynamically switches attention between the networks to respond to the environment and initiate tasks.[70] You make the meeting on time, even if you're frazzled and short of breath.

Theory of Mind

Our ability to function as a society requires us to understand and react appropriately to each other. Coordinated brain networks allow us to perceive other's viewpoints, beliefs, and to anticipate their actions. Called *theory of mind*, this ability helps us to intuit other's feelings, emotions, and intentions. It is a key element in being able to empathize, and comfort or help those around us.[71] Using theory of mind, we perceive our loved one's pain when he stubs his toe, or intuit his intentions by analyzing his facial expression and intonation.

Memory

Memory is critical to many types of cognition. Carrying on conversations, understanding the plot of a movie, or solving problems involves the ability to identify and remember key facts and data.

Memories are not housed in one area of the brain, but are laid down by linking sounds, aromas, and emotions with data, facts, and ideas stored in various areas of the brain.[72] This occurs in the hippocampus, near main white matter highways linking the networked areas. Neurons lay down memories by setting up these links. In the blink of an eye, catching a glimpse of a poster can recall a memory from our high school days; an aroma can bring back an emotionally charged moment or a longing for Hawaiian pizza; or a few measures of a song can bring back memories of hot afternoons sitting by the grill, eating steaks with your family. The experiences we remember are coalesced impressions registered by our brains of what we experienced at that moment in the past.

Retrieved memories often strengthen with frequent activation. We overwrite the neuronal memory pathway each time we recall and remember it.[73] Overwriting recalled memories can change or alter them over time. This is one of the reasons for differing memories between family members.

Brain Health Depends upon Good Blood Flow

A healthy brain requires good blood flow since it cannot store its own oxygen or energy. While only two percent of the body's mass, the brain consumes twenty percent of the body's energy.[74] As blood flows into the brain, it travels along smaller vessels until it reaches the capillaries. The sensitive architecture of the brain requires a tight blood-brain barrier to protect it from the toxic effects of many of the substances carried in the blood.

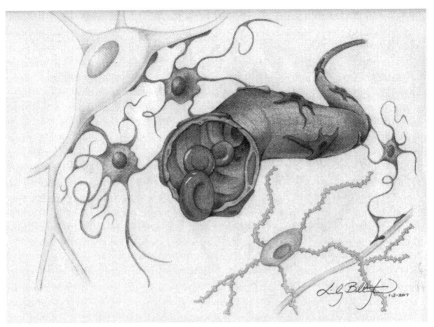

Figure 4 Neurovascular unit. Illustration by Lindsay J. Billington.

Recent studies discovered that the smallest blood vessels form a *neurovascular unit* consisting of specialized, tightly packed cells of the blood vessel walls; pericytes; glial cells called *astrocytes* that form connections between the blood vessel and the neurons; as well as neuronal projections called *axons* that work together to control blood flow. In a healthy unit, the cells of the blood vessel are tightly packed to control passage of water, fluids, proteins, glucose, and other substances.[75]

The close working relationship between the cells of the brain and those of the blood vessels is called *neurovascular coupling*. With increased neuronal activity, they call for more glucose through the astrocytes, which transmits the request to the cells lining the blood vessel.[76]

Our Brains Are Unique

Our physical attributes are genetically predetermined: short or tall, straight or curly hair, blue or brown eyes. However while most of our neurons have been laid down by the time we are born, the brain is still developing as glial cells proliferate and synapses grow and are strengthened by stimuli.[77] Glial cells wrap themselves around axonal bundles, insulating neural highways. Nutrition, home life, intellectual and emotional stimulation, as well as desires to learn and explore, all play a part in our brain's development.

Through experiences, learning, and stimulation, the areas utilized see synaptic growth, increased insulation, and become established, creating white matter highways connecting association areas. As we grow, we master movement and speech. Our perceptions of the physical world improve as our concrete reasoning makes sense of the world around us. Next, our abstract reasoning develops, helping us make plans and solve problems.

We inherit the basic capacities of our brains, such as musical or artistic ability, but the ultimate skill level achieved depends upon persistent hard work. Not everyone with great musical ability puts in the effort to master his talent. We have all met people with great intelligence that goes unused due to lack of ambition, while others with less talent, but greater motivation, achieve great things. Think of a box of LEGO® building blocks. Standard-sized pieces can produce a great variety of sculptures by the right artist.

Plasticity refers to the ability of our brain to adapt to the environment around us. How we react to our environment and its related stressors shapes our neuronal architecture. Neurons are not hard-wired connections, but multi-branching networks constantly shifting with the flow of input and thought processes. Choosing to learn a new language or how to play a musical instrument will stimulate certain areas to expand and develop. Deciding to forgive and not allow bitterness to grow; avoiding addictions to food or drugs; or acquiring new skills, such as learning how to play a guitar or how to speak Spanish, help shape our brains. Old ways of thinking and reacting can be changed and the brain re-patterned by how one chooses to think.

Do not be conformed to this world,
but be transformed by the renewal of your mind …
Romans 12:2

What Happens When Things Go Wrong in the Brain?

The networked, integrated brain rises above the sum of its parts. The brain's choreographed dance allows us to work together as a team, encourage and support one another, and create new products out of ordinary objects.

When there is sudden loss of cells in particular parts of the brain from stroke or traumatic brain injury, deficits occur. While the person might be able to recover some or most of the function over time, a degree of loss remains. However, with dementia, the cognitive deficits slowly build, with fits and starts. Here today, gone tomorrow, they appear intermittently or sporadically; hence the difficulty in perceiving dementia's presence in the early stages.

This pattern of intermittent difficulties could point to problems with sufficient levels of neurotransmitters—signals have difficulty getting through if the chemicals needed to jump the gap between neurons are missing. It could also indicate problems with the connectivity of the white matter highways that allow the associated areas and networks to operate effectively. Or, unresolved areas of inflammation create a breakdown of the blood-brain barrier, producing a cascade of problems that eventually lead to cellular loss.

High-level cognition and the ability to connect with others requires successful activation of the brain's many association areas for language, vision, and problem-solving, as well as the proper functioning of the higher level master networks. Failure in one area could impact far-flung areas. For example, if the thalamus, the key area for relaying signals for the brain's networks is impacted, deficits ranging from loss of consciousness to problems with memory retrieval could occur.

Commonalities of Most Diseases Causing Dementia

Dementia's Expression Varies Greatly from Person to Person

The variations in our cerebral structures lead to the unique expression of dementia. The exact nature of the deficits that develop with these diseases depend upon the part of the brain affected in relation to the health and structural development of that region. Areas, such as the hippocampus, which creates memories, may compensate for a while, but eventually the deficits will mushroom.

Some people with dementia do not recognize family members, develop paranoia, and become irritable or combative, while others experience severe speech difficulties, lose short-term memories, and can no longer learn. The variety from person to person in our brains and capacities affect the expression and pace of this disease, even among those with the same disease.[78]

My mother's dementia was a mixture of vascular cognitive impairment (VCI) and Alzheimer's. She had some of the characteristics of Alzheimer's, but not all of them. Her problems with memory pointed to Alzheimer's, while her periods of loss of function indicated VCI. The nature of the variable, plastic human brain, coupled with our limited understanding of our neurological system and lack of biomarkers to differentiate the disease(s) involved, explains why definitive diagnosis of dementia remains a challenge.

Symptoms Increase over Time

The diseases that cause dementia are neurodegenerative diseases—a breakdown of the central nervous system—which progressively worsen over time. Unlike a discrete event, such as a stroke or trauma, where deficits stabilize, neurodegenerative diseases produce increasing levels of disability. Lapses in memory and getting lost, bouts of confusion coupled with angry outbursts, and behavioral changes become more frequent and severe. Just as the family adjusted to Mom's *new normal*, she changed again.

Despite where dementia begins, the ripples from damaged and dying cells spread out to other areas of the brain. Cells in the brain's cortex are stacked in layers, as well as arranged in columns to form interconnected modules and units.[79] Like a wave spreading from the shore, degeneration follows well-established pathways until most of the brain is touched.

The rate of decline varies, depending upon which diseases are involved and the age of onset, along with an individual's unique factors. Early onset Alzheimer's (beginning before age sixty-five) may progress more quickly than late onset (any time after age sixty-four). Any trauma to the brain, such as an accident or operation, can exacerbate behaviors, push someone into the next stage, or bring the existence of dementia to light. Studies are still ongoing to understand why dementia progresses more rapidly in some individuals than in others.[80]

Overall, progression moves from mild to moderate to severe, if some other illness does not claim her life before she reaches the final stage. Not all people with dementia go through every stage. Many people usually contract dementia during old age and might also have heart disease, diabetes, cancer; or other ailments that could bring on death before the dementia progresses to its final stage. My friend Carol said that her mother never reached the final severe stage. A sudden medical emergency, making her mostly bed-bound and unable to feed herself, claimed her life within a two-week period.

Organic Denial—Anosognosia and Confabulation

Anosognosia is the loss of awareness of memory loss or presence of other neurological deficits. It had been assumed that the denial, so common with dementia, developed as a psychological coping mechanism. However, Dr. Robert Wilson of Rush University Medical Center in Chicago, Illinois, discovered some individuals could be unaware of any memory lapses up to two years before their diagnosis.[81]

Not only does your loved one lack awareness of her disease, leading her to deny any proof you show her, her brain will create explanations for the situations, called *confabulations*. These stories become so real to her that she cannot be persuaded they are not true. This can lead to outlandish accusations, such as your loved one believing you are sneaking into her house and stealing lost objects.

We constantly update our perceptions of reality by comparing what we expect or anticipate with actual results. Utilizing data from many sources, remembering them long enough to string together a picture of reality, we maintain an accurate perception of life occurring around us. Researchers believe structures in the center of the brain, front parts of the right temporal lobe, rear areas of the frontal lobes, in conjunction with parts of the parietal lobe at the top of the brain work together to create our perceptions of the world.[82] The degree of lack of awareness depends upon the extent of damage in these areas.[83]

In the beginning, your loved one may have perceived her memory lapses, only to have this awareness slip away as the degeneration deepens. Eventually, she will no longer be able to react to her memory lapses as she descends into the more severe stages of dementia.[84]

Even if our loved one has anosognosia, her active reasoning areas are still trying to make sense of events. She will latch onto bits and pieces, sometimes long dormant, to fabricate a plausible scenario—the confabulation storyline—which becomes her reality.

⸙

During a meeting with their mother's nursing home administrator, my friend Carol and her brother, David, were told, "Your mom said she's getting married next week."

They looked at each other in amazement.

"Does this mean something to you?"

Carol said, "Next week is my mother's anniversary."

The administrator added with a smile, "She said she's getting married next week, but she doesn't know to whom."

Carol suspected one of the many calendars might have jogged her mother's memory enough to recognize the date related to a wedding. Not recalling the rest of the facts, Mary just knew she was going to be married next week. Indeed she had, many years before.

Some days, the links all connect and memories reflect the whole story. Some days, we can see bits and pieces of their lives in their stories. Even when every fact does not quite line up, we can still honor them and their lives by listening and affirming. Sometimes when my mother came out with statements like Mary's, I would nod and smile.

When dementia begins to affect any part of this interactive network, our loved one's ability to accurately perceive the world begins to falter. In the beginning, she may lapse into unawareness and storytelling, eventually living in a world that no longer corresponds to reality.[85] Her cognitive difficulties have rendered her unable to correctly perceive our world (her theory of mind ability has been altered).

Great tension results when we do not go along with our loved one's explanations and try to change her perceptions. To help her cope, we need to meet her in her world. We can empathize and try to come alongside to seek solutions. Some days, we are able to redirect, to move on to a solution, and provide the emotional support she needs.

The stories created to explain her reality can center around one person whom she blames for all her troubles. Sometimes, redirecting or trying to find creative solutions might work. If the accusations are caused by other issues that can be resolved, you might be able to move forward. However, if she sees you as the cause, even if you helped her greatly in the past, and her hostility persists, you might have to back away for a time. There might be someone else in the family she trusts who can become the primary caregiver. We will explore handling anosognosia as a caregiver in greater depth in Chapter 6: The Middle-Moderate Stages.

When a loved one becomes a stranger and then your enemy, you can continue to commit him to the Lord's care. Romans 12:14-21 instructs us to love our enemies and do good to them. If we can extend gracious love to our enemies, we can do the same for our family and friends who might treat us as enemies. Doing good to him despite his accusations, patiently handling the insults, seeking to minister to him in his need when he is unlovable can be accomplished with God's help.

Do not be overcome by evil,
but overcome evil with good.
Romans 12:21

They Do Not Lose Their Humanity

All of us are created in the image of God. Whether we are highly functioning or profoundly disabled, we remain persons. We still need to relate to others, give and receive love, and be useful.

While living in her first unit at the nursing home, Mary decided the other residents in wheelchairs needed to be pushed about the facility. Carol, in talking about her mother's time in the nursing home said, "The only problem they had with her was that she wanted to help people. She would buy Christmas presents for people. She wanted to push people around in their wheelchairs and they didn't want to go. That's when they moved her out of the Alzheimer's unit since it had the more critical patients." Carol's mother wanted to be useful.

My mother, a registered dietician, while in her earlier stages, gladly advised the Sienna Crest staff on healthy eating habits and lifestyles. We all want to do what we can to help.

As a relational being, our loved one needs our love and respect. "A new commandment I give to you, that you love one another: just as I have loved you, you also are to love one another" (John 13:34). God's commandment to love one another does not end when dementia appears. It increases the necessity. God loves her more than we do. He will guide us in how to help her.

The next section, building upon what we have learned about the brain's structure and function, will tie together the disease progression with changes in the brain.

Brain Changes with the Four Diseases

Let's recap the main characteristics for the four major dementia diseases:

Alzheimer's disease (AD): Begins with memory problems accompanied by slow, steady deterioration in planning, reasoning, mathematical ability, orientation (date, time, place), and speech.

Vascular cognitive impairment (VCI): Occurs in step-like progression with some stabilization, with varying symptoms depending upon where the brain damage occurred, and may follow AD progression.

Frontotemporal dementia (FTD): Begins either with behavioral, speech, or emotional problems depending upon where the degeneration begins, while memory problems usually occur later.

Lewy body dementia (LBD): Begins with acting out dreams (REM behavior disorder), hallucinations, and difficulties with problem-solving, planning, and problems with maintaining body states such as steady blood pressure.

Alzheimer's Disease (AD)

With Alzheimer's disease, decreased production of neurotransmitters accompanies synaptic destruction and nerve cell death. Shrinking cells, with fewer synapses and neurotransmitters, struggle to perform, eventually die and are absorbed by the body.

The progression seems to work backwards, starting with most recent memories and skills lost first. Called *retrogenesis* by Dr. Reisberg of New York University (see Chapter 2: Dementia Basics),

Alzheimer's progression appears to walk backward from adulthood to childhood to infancy. Dr. Tam Cummings, a gerontologist and dementia expert from Texas detailed the spread of Alzheimer's disease through the brain for the classic patient.

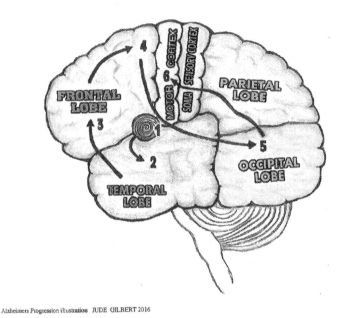

Alzheimers Progression illustration JUDE GILBERT 2016

Figure 5 Dr. Cummings' typical sequence for Alzheimer's progression through the brain.[86] Illustration by Jude Gilbert.

1 The first symptoms usually begin with memory issues since this disease typically begins in the center of the brain near the *hippocampus.*

2 The disease then spreads to the front of the *temporal lobes,* affecting speech.

3 In the *frontal lobes,* it affects reasoning, thinking, and impulse control.

4 It continues to move along the *cerebral cortex,* the outer layers of the brain affecting analytical thought and movement.

5 Passing through the temporal lobes, it impacts the *occipital lobes,* the main visual area.

6 Eventually, it spreads to the *parietal areas* affecting sensory perception, and ability to identify temperature, and pain sensations.

When dementia begins with damage to the hippocampus, our loved one will not remember recent events, such as what she bought at the store that day; she might not be able to access her internal maps to remember where her home is in relation to her favorite grocery store. Additionally, damage to the nearby hypothalamus impacts her internal circadian rhythm. She begins to lose track of the time of day, such as thinking it's time to get up even if it's the middle of the night.[87]

At first, this disorientation usually begins with losing maps—getting lost in familiar areas. Next, she loses touch with the time she inhabits—for example, understanding she is eighty years old and remembering her past. She might think she is thirty and raising her family. Not able to place herself in context, she loses connection to the time signature of her memories.

Lost memories are a failure of the brain's networks to connect the dots to recall a person or an event. In the beginning, the networks fail to link recent events, but already established memories can still be retrieved. Loss of recent memory can lead to repeatedly asking the same question or retelling the same story in a short period of time—this is called *perseveration*. Eventually, mostly the strongest memories remain. As our loved one's memories dwindle, she might seem to move back in time. The process varies from day to day or hour to hour—on good days a memory can be retrieved that appeared lost the week before—as the ability to recall decreases over time.[88]

The amygdala, closely connected to the hippocampus, is also affected early on in the disease and atrophies at about the same rate as the hippocampus. As Alzheimer's advances, learned controls that helped navigation of his social world erode and your loved one can begin to say and do things totally out of character. When the amygdala and areas of the frontal lobes atrophy, his anxiety lessens, along with his ability to control his impulses.[89] Internal filters, developed over decades, may have eroded past the point for him to respond graciously to difficult situations.

Language difficulties appear when the temporal lobes are

damaged. Sudden cursing in inappropriate situations also points to damage in the left temporal lobe. She can no longer remember how to verbalize her feelings, but she can still say the expressive words housed in the right temporal lobe.[90]

Not being able to recognize friends and family is associated with loss in the facial recognition areas of the temporal lobes along with damage to the visual system in the occipital lobes.[91] To some, most faces look unfamiliar. To others, most faces can look familiar even if they cannot recognize them.

Mom and I were in line at the local coffee shop, getting our favorite lattes with scones. Mom looked back at the couple behind us with a toddler in the stroller.

"They go to our church," she said, smiling broadly at them.

"No, they don't," I replied just before I ordered our drinks. when she insisted, I nodded my head and watched the barista brew our coffees.

I was beginning to understand that trying to convince her people around us were not friends from church was a lost cause. I smiled at the couple and helped my friendly mother to a table by the front window.

The ability to focus on a particular speaker in a noisy environment becomes more difficult with Alzheimer's. Studies have shown people with Alzheimer's compensate for a while, increasing activation in the usual areas of the brain as well as utilizing other parts of the brain to focus on one speaker in a crowded room.[92] Eventually, the brain loses the ability to decrease background noise and enhance target sounds, making crowded areas torturous for your loved one.

Damage to the temporal lobes where it connects with the parietal lobes has been linked to a theory of mind deficit. They cannot perceive other's feelings and thoughts.[93] This, combined with a lack of control due to frontal lobe deficits, can lead to egocentric, self-centered behavior.

⌘

One of my nieces reflected on the changes in her grandmother. "Before, she would rise at the crack of dawn and start reading her Bible. She gave us whatever we wanted—hot chocolate, pancakes. She really doted on us, talked to us for hours, and told us stories. Those memories are what I really treasure. So now, for her to not talk to us, or snap at us, or disregard us as if we weren't there was a mean thing for her to do. I don't remember completely what she said. It was a shocker for us. That was hard and part of the grieving process."

⌘

Damage to the frontal lobes not only erodes self-control, it impacts analytical and mathematical reasoning. When this area is damaged along with the areas for mathematical reasoning in the parietal lobes, his ability to manage finances, to plan, or to anticipate events degrades. It also impacts the ability to complete the steps of a task in the right order.[94] This can begin to happen early on and explains why he has trouble completing projects and might start avoiding activities he used to enjoy. Decreased reasoning ability means he might not understand that fall means cooler temperatures and that he will need warmer clothing.

Another form of perseveration (repeating an action, phrase, or question over and over) arises from damage to the frontal lobes.[95] In the thinking, reasoning parts of the frontal lobes, the brain selects and initiates the next step or action. When the brain cannot focus attention, or retain the event in working memory, perseveration occurs.[96] In time, if the frontal lobes have difficulty switching tasks or stopping the loop, it repeats it. Being stuck in a loop can occur if the brain's ability to dynamically switch from one activity to the next is impaired. Sometimes redirection, distraction, or trying to switch focus on another task helps break the cycle.

It has been discovered that people with Alzheimer's disease

have a disruption in the default mode network (DMN) hindering memory recall. Conversely, the salience network (SN) becomes more active.[97] The disrupted DMN can lead to loss of memory as well as greater difficulty recalling personal family history, at the same time the enhanced SN increases responsiveness to emotions expressed by others.[98] For example, while your loved one might not be able to state who you are to her, she will innately understand she can trust you.[99] While she might not remember I am her daughter, she can feel if I am irritable or rushed. She did not choose to forget I was her daughter.

When the damage begins to impact the occipital lobes where the brain interprets the signals from the eyes, she will not be able to identify the images her eyes see. She might not recognize your face or a chair, or could believe a shiny, waxed floor is too wet to step on.[100] The brain might create visual hallucinations, so she sees people lurking in the shadows and thinks intruders are coming.

While my friend Carol was living with her mother, Mary would tell the landlord to send a plumber since she had seen a leak in the basement. Eventually, Carol had to tell the management company to only take calls from her (Carol) as there was no leak in the basement. Mary also called Carol at work to tell her their dog was bleeding. When she arrived home, she could see his belly was red from scratching, but he was not bleeding. Mary's brain was having trouble interpreting what her eyes were seeing.

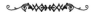

As the disease moves into the parietal lobes, she will not be able to identify the location of pains or itches, nor be able to identify hot or cold.[101] Damage to the right parietal lobe impairs the ability to judge distances, making it hard to navigate steps and uneven surfaces.[102]

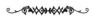

Toward the end, when Mom would scrunch her face up, the aide would ask her, "Where does it hurt, Edith?"

She would look at the aide blankly or sometimes shake her head, but we knew she was experiencing pain somewhere.

The aide worked through the most likely places—it was usually the corn on the ball of her right foot. We made sure the corn was cut back, applied lotion, and gave her a massage.

Mom could no longer tell us where it hurt.

Vascular Cognitive Impairment (VCI)

While for many years it was believed that cognitive impairment was due to blocked or ruptured blood vessels, dementia may begin with a breakdown of the neurovascular unit.

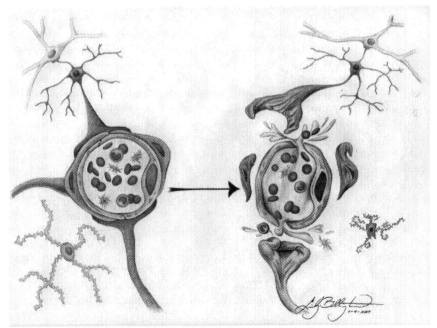

Figure 6 Breakdown of the NVU. Illustration by Lindsay J. Billington.

The blood-brain barrier is compromised when the tight junctions between the cells lining the blood vessels loosen and separate, allowing fluids and toxins to flood the fragile brain matrix. Inflammation plays a part in the breakdown of the blood-brain barrier.[103] Over time, as more areas are affected faster than can be repaired, nearby brain cells become damaged or incapacitated. Research established impaired blood flow to brain regions eventually produces cognitive impairment.[104] People who have experienced strokes might develop dementia. However, the emergence of dementia without documented strokes points to compromised blood flow.

Dementia is more likely when the brain is not able to resolve pockets of inflammation and return these areas to normal functioning. This has been documented with both Alzheimer's disease and VCI, one of the many ways these two diseases intersect.[105]

The ability of interconnected neuronal and blood vessel cells to communicate decreases with age. Areas needing greater blood flows are less able to get their needs met. Different brain regions have different energy needs. For example, the cerebellum, with fewer glial cells per neurons, has lower energy requirements than the active hippocampus with its larger concentration of glial cells. The greater energy requirements of areas such as the hippocampus could be the reason dementia often begins in these areas when blood flow cannot satisfy the cellular demands.[106] The areas at greater risk due to decreased blood supply are the very areas impacted earlier with Alzheimer's disease.

Vascular cognitive impairment (VCI) produces a sudden onset of varying symptoms, depending upon the areas affected. A person with VCI seems to stabilize after each incident, but never quite returns to her previous cognitive levels. This differs from the slow, steady downhill slide of Alzheimer's. Her symptoms will vary greatly depending upon the location of the affected areas: she may develop weakness, problems walking or maintaining balance, tremors, trouble seeing or hearing, or slurred speech. She might begin expressing inappropriate emotions. She might be able to understand speech, but be unable to retrieve her words, impeding her ability to respond verbally.

When there is a mixture of vascular dementia and Alzheimer's, there is a slow, gradual decline between episodes. The trajectory can be similar to the "typical" Alzheimer's path, along with deficits that appear more abruptly. The hallmark of VCI is punctuated decline over time. The progression seems to go in bursts, accelerating then slowing, only to advance again.

Frontotemporal Dementia (FTD)

While frontotemporal dementia has some brain atrophy, the resemblance to Alzheimer's stops there. Since the disease begins with the frontal lobes (this type is called behavior variant FTD–bvFTD) or temporal lobes, memory is usually not the primary symptom in the beginning. Instead, a person with FTD will show personality changes, develop antisocial behaviors, stop showing emotions, or have great difficulty speaking.[107]

Frontal Lobes—Behavior Variant FTD (bvFTD)

The loss of ability to sacrifice short-term pleasures for future rewards shows up early in bvFTD, leading to antisocial behaviors. The ability of the prefrontal cortex in the frontal lobe to control behavior by reasoning through a situation, utilizing memories of learned responses, current sensory data, and emotional input is impaired. A person with bvFTD might shoplift, not understand appropriate dress or social interactions, or begin swearing.

Researchers have discovered that someone with bvFTD has reduced function in the salience network (SN), which impedes his ability to respond appropriately.[108] This is called *emotional blunting*. He has a more difficult time understanding the emotions and intentions of others.[109] Less able to understand the sorrow or fear of those around him, he appears self-centered and egotistical. The inappropriate behavior has also been linked to a theory of mind deficit with a person's inability to inhibit his actions for the benefit of others.[110] Conversely, the default mode network is enhanced leading to greater artistic ability in some.[111]

A piano teacher who enjoyed giving lessons at home was diagnosed with FTD at the age of forty-eight. She lost interest in her husband and teenage daughter, preferring to eat alone in front of the TV, and refusing to help her daughter find a prom dress. When her husband was in the hospital recovering from cancer surgery, she did not visit him and told her daughter to stop crying like a baby. She stated, "I know I'm supposed to feel something when they cry, but I just don't." Antidepressants and counselling were not able to help her regain her ability to emotionally connect with her family. She still played the piano, even while living in a care facility.[112]

The frontal lobes initiate and control movements. He can become overactive and wander or pace as he has greater difficulty shifting from one action to another. This might cause perseveration—repeating the same actions or phrases over and over. He may develop complex rituals, obsessions, and repetitive behaviors such as clapping, tapping, singing, or whistling.[113]

Behavior variant FTD also impacts the thalamus, a key part of the center of the brain and white matter highway for major brain networks, particularly the salience network (SN). BvFTD behaviors can result from a mixture of impaired salience network (SN) deficits in areas of the frontal lobes, along with possible disruptions to the brain's networks due to problems with the thalamus. Impairment in the thalamus and corresponding network has been associated with impulse control and decision-making difficulties.[114]

Decreased functional connectivity between networks results in lessened response to pain as signals have a harder time getting through. Your loved one might not perceive he is overheating, forget to remove his jacket, or not feel the pain from the swelling and bruising caused by a fall.[115] For some people, sudden changes in sense of humor and less self-consciousness caused by deterioration in the connecting fibers in the thalamus can be early signs of this disease.[116]

If damage occurs in the nearby hypothalamus, which controls eating patterns, he might start binge eating particular foods and refuse to eat other types of foods.[117] With an impaired hypothalamus, he might not sense internal cues telling him to stop eating. Many people with bvFTD will overeat and prefer sweeter food, leading to weight gain.[118]

These causes produce varying symptoms dependent upon the degree of impairment in particular areas. A loved one might have developed binge eating while another might make inappropriate gestures in public.[119]

FTD Beginning with the Temporal Lobes

Many of the fundamentals of speech are housed in the left temporal lobe, just beside the left ear, where we assign meanings to words and formulate sentences. This is where we store long-term and autobiographical memories about ourselves, dates, and places. Due to the problems with language, this variation of FTD may also be called "primary progressive aphasia" or "semantic dementia" (many names exist for the variation seen with FTD).[120]

When FTD begins in the left temporal lobes, a person will not only have trouble finding words but also lose the understanding of what the words mean. Atrophy eventually spreads to the hippocampus and amygdala, affecting memory and emotions. As the disease progresses, it eventually encompasses the frontal lobes, and then the right temporal lobe.[121]

The ability to embed emotion in speech and actions comes from the right temporal lobe. In some instances, dementia may start in the right lobe. This leads to increased loss of empathy, flatness of emotion, and to the inability to understand other's emotions and add emotional content to our speech and singing.

FTD Progression

As with the other types of dementias, patients will exhibit some of the symptoms, depending upon which lobes are affected, as well as which layers of the lobes. Some diseases begin in the outer cortical areas, while others arise in deeper areas of the impacted lobes.

During the mild stage, the disease often affects one lobe with fairly slow progression. Usually, damage does not begin in the other lobes until the middle stages when progression accelerates. Some people who begin with behavioral problems (if it started in the frontal lobes) might lose their ability to communicate as the disease moves to the temporal lobes in the middle stages. If the disease moves into the deeper areas of the brain, some people might have problems with motor coordination, cognition, and learning. Eventually, as the disease spreads, their movements might resemble the tremors, rigidity, and slow movements of Parkinson's. By the severe stage, they will be totally dependent on help for all activities, even losing the ability to swallow.[122]

Lewy Body Dementia (LBD)

With Lewy body dementia, alpha-synuclein protein clumps, called Lewy bodies, develop in neurons and glial cells in the brainstem, key structures in the center of the brain, certain areas of the frontal lobes, hippocampus, and the occipital lobes.[123] These areas have decreased neurotransmitter levels and cerebral blood flow.

Episodes of loss of consciousness have been linked to problems in the thalamic area, a critical white matter highway relay station for the brain. Some researchers believe sudden changes of awareness, including abrupt loss of consciousness, occur as a result of damage in the thalamus.[124]

These areas are associated with a decrease in a key enzyme for the production of the neurotransmitter, acetylcholine. This is the reason why Alzheimer's drugs that decrease the breakdown of acetylcholine work well for many people with LBD.[125] When neurons have decreased neurotransmitter levels, their signals have a harder time crossing the gap between the dendrites and nearby axons, eventually leading to dendrite loss. These deficits force the brain's networks to find other routes to connect thought-processing areas.[126]

Another study found problems with switching out of the default mode network (DMN) to focus attention or solve problems, and theorized that the failure to deactivate the DMN points to difficulties to dynamically focus attention when needed.[127] This could be a contributing factor to the day-by-day, sometimes hour-by-hour, changes in cognitive abilities. The roller-coaster experience, where they can bounce from severe-to-mild-to-moderate in a short period of time, makes it hard to keep up with current demands or plan. Some people can function fairly well for part of the day, be unable to stay awake for the rest, be greatly confused the next morning, and then rebound the next day. LBD does not follow the gradual decline as seen with Alzheimer's.

Decreases in neurotransmitters were discovered in the occipital lobes possibly creating the visual hallucinations.[128] Impaired circulation was also found in this area.[129] Compromised blood flow was also identified in the temporal and parietal regions—key neural network areas.[130] Studies found resting-state networks that connect to the occipital areas had impaired connectivity. Having trouble receiving incoming signals and relaying analysis of the inputs appears to be a contributing factor for visual problems.[131]

The thalamus has also been identified as the key center for neural processing during sleep.[132] Many people who develop REM sleep behavior disorders (RBD—physically acting out dreams) go on to develop LBD.[133] The disruptions in parts of the thalamus might contribute to the sleep disturbances.

People with LBD can also develop movement disorders, similar to Parkinson's, due to connectivity issues with the sensory-motor network. A link was discovered between the disruptions for the sensory-motor networks and connected areas in the thalamus that were key components for cognition that could also be causing fluctuations.[134]

Lewy bodies also occur with Parkinson's, but arise in the brain stem instead of the cortex. Parkinson's leads to movement problems as the substantia nigra in the brain stem are affected. Some individuals with Parkinson's eventually develop dementia.[135]

Taking a quick peek under the hood helps us grasp more fully that our loved one's words and actions might be beyond her conscious control. We need to remember what our loved one was like before the disease(s) impacted her behavior, and not forget it's the dementia talking.

The interconnected brain systems can stutter and falter if some parts weaken or fail. For example, low neurotransmitter levels could impair a cognitive network. Understanding this helps explain why my mother's memory seemed so sporadic. One day, she recognized me; the next day, not so much. Some weeks, she remembered to get ready for church, and then she would forget. Just because our loved one cannot remember today does not mean she will not remember tomorrow—she might or she might not.

Additionally, even if our loved one has deficits in one area, that does not mean she has deficits in all areas. While she might not be able to speak, she might still be able to read and write. Even though my mother, a registered dietician, could no longer recall the essential amino acids, she could still reach out to comfort a neighbor. So, we had to let her do as much for herself as possible. If it's not working that day, we move on; if she succeeds, we have a good day to look back on. Every day is a new day.

Part 2, Chapters 4 through 7 will cover the major issues, ways of thinking, and helps for navigating the journey with our loved one. Despite the differences between the many diseases that cause dementia, everyone experiences many of the issues.

---

[42] Professor Ken Ashwell, *The Brain Book: Development, Function, Disorder, Health* (Buffalo, NY: Firefly Books, 2012), p 78.

43 R Douglas Fields, PhD, *The Other Brain: From Dementia to Schizophrenia, How New Discoveries about the Brain Are Revolutionizing Medicine and Science* (New York: Simon & Schuster, 2009), pp 22-23, 261.

44 Ibid., pp 35, 44-45, and 65.

45 Ashwell, p 18.

46 Ibid., pp 30-31.

47 Ibid., pp 32-33.

48 Regina Bailey, "Hippocampus." https://www.thoughtco.com/hippocampus-anatomy-373221. Accessed 9/9/2017.

49 Jack Fincher, *The Human Body: The Brain: Mystery of Matter and Mind.* (New York: Torstar Books, 1984), p 92.

50 Rita Carter, Susan Aldridge, Martyn Page, and Steve Parker, *The Human Brain Book* (China: Dorling Kindersley Ltd., 2014), p 162.

51 Benjamin J Kraus, Mark P Brandon, Robert J Robinson II, Michael A Connerney, Michael E Hasselmo, and Howard Eichenbaum (2015). "During running in place, grid cells integrate elapsed time and distance run." *Neuron.* 88(3):578-589. www.ncbi.nlm.nih.gov/pubmed/26539893. Accessed 11/28/2016.

52 Ashwell, p 244.

53 Ibid., p 187. And H Braak, E Braak, D Yilmazer and J Bohl (1996), "Functional anatomy of human hippocampal formation and related structures." *Journal of Child Neurology.* 11(4):265-275. www.ncbi.nlm.nih.gov/pubmed/8807415. Accessed 5/16/2016.

54 Ashwell, p 144.

55 Fincher, p 30.

56 Ibid., p 32. And Katherine P Rankin, PhD, "Chapter 15. Altered Relationships: Adapting to Emotions and Behavior," in Gary Radin and Lisa Radin (eds.), *What If It's Not Alzheimer's?: A Caregiver's Guide to Dementia,* 3rd ed. (Amherst, NY: Prometheus Books, 2014), p 238.

57 Ashwell, p 20.

58 Rossor in Radin and Radin, pp 30-31. And Ashwell, p 20.

59 Carter et al., p 157.

60 Ashwell, p 164.

61 Cummings, pp 77-78.

62 Carter et al., p 92.

63 Ashwell, p 193.

64 Ibid., p 157. And Carter et al., pp 120-121.

65 Cummings, p 83.

66 Dr. Kevin McGrew, "The Brain as a Network: Focusing Your Network" (December 22, 2011). www.creativitypost.com/psychology/the_brain_as_a_network_focusing_your_network. Accessed 11/30/2015.

[67] SL Bressler and V Menon (2010). "Large-scale brain networks in cognition: emerging methods and principles." *Trends in Cognitive Sciences* 14:277-290. Scottbarrykaufman.com/wp-content/uploads/2013/08/Bressler_Large-Scale_Brain_ 10.pdf. Accessed 11/30/2015.

[68] Ibid.

[69] McGrew.

[70] Ibid.

[71] Ashwell, pp 208-210.

[72] Petersen, p 31.

[73] Carter et al., p 162.

[74] Ibid., p 45.

[75] DB Stanimirovic and A Friedman (2012). "Pathophysiology of the neurovascular unit: disease cause or consequence?" *Journal of Cerebral Blood Flow & Metabolism* 32:1207-1221. Published online March 7, 2012. www. ncbi.nlm.nih. gov/pubmed/22395208. Accessed 9/10/2017.

[76] Ibid. And KM Dunn and MT Nelson (2014). "Neurovascular signaling in the brain and the pathological consequences of hypertension." *American Journal of Physiology Heart and Circulatory Physiology*. 306(1):H1-H14. www.ncbi. nlm. nih.gov/pmc/articles/PMC3920149/ Accessed 11/6/2015.

[77] Andrew Koob, *The Root of Thought: Unlocking Glia—The Brain Cell that Will Help Us Sharpen Our Wits, Heal Injury, and Treat Brain Disease* (Upper Saddle River, NJ: Pearson Education, Inc., 2009), p 69.

[78] Alzheimer's Association, "Stages of Alzheimer's." www.alz.org/alzheimers_ disease_stages_of_alzheimers.asp. Accessed 10/28/2016.

[79] Rodney J Douglas, Misha A Mahowald and Kevan AC Martin, "Microarchitecture of Neocortical Columns," in *Brain Theory: Biological Basis and Computational Principles*, A Aertsen and V Braitenberg, eds. (Amsterdam: Elsevier, 1996), pp 75, 81. And Roger A Barker, BA, MSS, MRCP, *Neuroscience: An Illustrated Guide* (New York: Ellis Horwood, 1991), p 218.

[80] A search of pubmed (a federal database of research articles found at www.ncbi. nlm.nih.gov/pubmed) showed many studies found increased progression with earlier onset, for example--G Tosto, M Gasparini, AM Brickman, F Letteri, R Renie, P Piscopo, G Talarico, M Canevelli, A Confaloni, and G Bruno (2015). "Neuropsychological predictors of rapidly progressive Alzheimer's disease." *Acta Neurologica Scandinavica*. 132(6):417-422. www.ncbi.nlm.nih. gov/pubmed/ 25903925. Some did not find a correlation with earlier onset—H Grønning, Rahmani, J Gyllenborg, RB Dessau, and P Høgh (2012). "Does Alzheimer's disease with early onset progress faster than with late onset? A case-control study of clinical progression and cerebrospinal fluid biomarkers." *Dementia and Geriatric Cognitive Disorders*. 33(2-3):111-117. www.ncbi.nlm.

nih.gov/pubmed /22508568. Interestingly, one study found while dementia is less likely among those with higher education, once diagnosed, the disease appears to progress more rapidly —H Cho, S Jeon, C Kim, BS Ye, GH Kim, Y Noh, HJ Kim, CW Yoon, YJ Kim, JH Kim, SE Park, ST Kim, JM Lee, SJ Kang, MK Suh, J Chin, DL Na, DR Kang, and SW Seo (2015). "Higher education affects accelerated cortical thinning in Alzheimer's disease: a 5-year preliminary longitudinal study." *International Psychogeriatrics.* 27(1):111-120. www.ncbi.nlm.nih.gov/pubmed/25226082. Accessed 6/2/2016.

81 RS Wilson, PA Boyle, L Yu, LL Barnes, J Sytsma, AS Buchman, DA Bennett, and JA Schneider (2015). "Temporal course and pathologic basis of unawareness of memory loss in dementia." *Neurology* 10.1212 published online August 26, 2015. www.neurology.org/content/85/11/984. Accessed 9/9/2017.

82 L Pia, M Neppi-Modona, R Ricci, and A Berti, "The Anatomy of Anosognosia for Hemiplegia: A Meta-Analysis." *Cortex* 40(2)367-377. www.sciencedirect. com/ science/article/pii/S001094520870131X. Accessed 12/21/2015.

83 Treatment Advocacy Center, "The Anatomical Basis of Anosognosia-Backgrounder." Updated May 24, 2016. http://www.treatmentadvocacycenter. org/ fixing-the-system/features-and-news/3080-the-anatomical-basis-of-anosognosia. Accessed 9/9/2017.

84 Shelly Webb, "Two Words Every Dementia Caregiver Should Know." Excellent article on anosognosia and confabulation. http://www.intentionalcaregiver. com/ two-key-words/. Accessed 9/9/2017.

85 Ibid.

86 Cummings, p 77.

87 John Zeisel, PhD, *I'm Still Here: A New Philosophy of Alzheimer's Care* (New York: Avery: Penguin Group USA, 2010), p 76.

88 Cummings, pp 65-66.

89 SP Poulin, M.D., R Dautoff, B.S., JC Morris, M.D., L Feldman-Barrett, Ph.D., and BC Dickerson, M.D. (2011). "Amygdala atrophy is prominent in early Alzheimer's disease and relates to symptom severity." *Psychiatry Research.* 194(1):7-13. www.ncbi.nlm.nih.gov/pmc/articles/PMC3185127/. Accessed 11/2/2015. This study was conducted as part of the Alzheimer's disease Neuroimaging Initiative (ADNI).

90 Cummings, p 78.

91 Alzheimer's Society, "The brain and dementia: 4. Dementia symptoms and areas of the brain." www.alzheimers.org.uk/Info/20073/how_dementia_progresses/99/ the_brain_and_dementia/4. Accessed 9/10/2017. Face recognition area is housed in the right temporal lobe. See Carter et al., p 84.

92 HL Golden, JL Agustus, JC Goll, LE Downey, CJ Mummery, JM Schott, SJ Crutch, and JD Warren (2015). "Functional neuroanatomy of auditory

scene analysis in Alzheimer's disease." *NeuroImage: Clinical* 7:699-708. Published online February 28, 2015. www.sciencedirect.com/science/article/ pii/S221315821 5000376. Accessed 12/8/2015. And S Kamourieh, R Braga, R Leech and R Wise (2015). "Dementia and the cocktail party (P1.205)" *Neurology* 84(14):Supplement P1.205. Published online April 8, 2015. www. neurology.org/content/84/14_ Supplement/P1.205. Accessed 9/10/2017.

93   R Le Bouc, P Lenfant, X Delbeuck, L Ravasi, F Lebert, F Seman, and F Pasquier (2012). "My belief or yours? Differential theory of mind deficits in frontotemporal dementia and Alzheimer's disease." *Brain* 135(Pt 10):3026-3038. www.ncbi.nlm. nih.gov/pubmed/23065791. Accessed 5/13/2016.

94   Zeisel, p 69.

95   Harriet Hodgson, "The Perseveration (Getting Stuck) That Comes With Memory Disease" (2006). www.ezinearticles.com/?The-Perseveration-(Getting-Stuck)-That-Comes-With-Memory-Disease&id=391287. Accessed 9/10/2017.

96   Cláudia Guarda, Ana Silvestre, Élia Baeta, and Miguel Viana Baptista (2008). P3-138: Perseveration in Alzheimer's disease and vascular dementia. *Alzheimer's & Dementia* 4(4):Supplement T560. www.alzheimersanddementia.com/ article/ S1552-5260(08)01863-3/abstract. Accessed 9/10/2017.

97   Alison Kevan, "Dementia and the distinct patterns of brain disorganization." dementiaresearchfoundation.org.au/blog/dementia-and-distinct-patterns-brain-disorganisation. Accessed 9/10/2017.

98   Michael Hornberger, "Brain network dysfunction in frontotemporal dementia." http://www.ftdtalk.org/brain-network-dysfunction-in-frontotemporal-dementia/. Accessed 9/10/2017.

99   Ibid.

100 Cummings, p 82.

101 Ibid., p 83.

102 Alzheimer's Society.

103 MA Lopez-Ramirez, D Wu, G Pryce, JE Simpson, A Reijerkerk, J King-Robson, O Kay, HE de Vries, MC Hirst, B Sharrack, D Baker, DK Male, GJ Michael, and IA Romero (2014). "MicroRNA-155 negatively affects blood-brain barrier function during neuroinflammation." *The FASEB Journal* 28(6):2551-2565. www.fasebj.org/content/28/6/2551.abstract. Accessed 1/11/2016. Related news release – Federation of American Societies for Experimental Biology, "Why inflammation leads to a leaky blood-brain barrier: MicroRNA-155." www.eurekalert.org/pub_releases/2014-06/foas-wil060214.php. Accessed 1/11/2016.

104 A Ruitenberg, T den Heijer, SL Bakker, JC van Swieten, PJ Koudstaal, A Hofman, and MM Breteler (2005). "Cerebral hypoperfusion and clinical onset of dementia: the Rotterdam Study." *Annals of Neurology* 57(6):789-794.

www.ncbi.nlm.nih.gov/pubmed/15929050. Accessed 1/11/2016. And Z Jing, C Shi, L Zhu, Y Xiang, P Chen, Z Xiong, W Li, Y Ruan, and L Huang (2015). "Chronic cerebral hypoperfusion induces vascular plasticity and hemodynamics but also neuronal degeneration and cognitive impairment." *Journal of Cerebral Blood Flow & Metabolism* 35(8):1249-1259. www.ncbi. nlm.nih.gov/pubmed/ 25853908. Accessed 9/10/2017.

105 LV Androsova, NM Miklaĭlova, SA Zozulia, AM Dupin, GA Rassadina, NV Lavrent'eva, and TP Kluishnik (2013). [Inflammatory markers in Alzheimer's disease and vascular dementia]. *Zh Nevrol Psikhiatr Im SS Korsakova* 113(2):49-53. [Russian.] www.ncbi.nlm.nih.gov/pubmed/23528583. Accessed 1/13/2016. The inability to resolve cerebral inflammation was also highlighted by X Wang, M Zhu, E Hjorth, V Cortés-Toro, H Eyjolfsdottir, C Graff, I Nennesmo, J Palmblad, M Eriksdotter, K Sambamurti, JM Fitzgerald, CN Serhan, AC Granholm, and M Schultzberg (2015). "Resolution of inflammation is altered in Alzheimer's disease." *Alzheimers & Dementia.* 11(1):40-50. www.alzheimersanddementia. com/article/S1552-5260(14)00030-2/abstract. Accessed 12/16/2015.

106 JC de la Torre (2012). "Cardiovascular risk factors promote brain hypoperfusion leading to cognitive decline and dementia." *Cardiovascular Psychiatry and Neurology* 2012(Article ID 367516), 15 pages. www.hindawi.com/journals/ cpn/ 2012/367516/. Accessed 1/11/2016.

107 Rossor in Radin and Radin, p 33.

108 J Zhou, MD Greicius, ED Gennatas, ME Growdon, JY Jang, GD Rabinovici, JH Kramer, M Weiner, BL Miller, and WW Seeley (2010). "Divergent network connectivity changes in behavoural variant frontotemporal dementia and Alzheimer's disease." *Brain* 133:1352-1367. www.ncbi.nlm.nih.gov/pubmed/ 20140145. Accessed 9/10/2017.

109 C Cerami, A Dodich, N Canessa, C Credspi, A Marcone, F cortese, G Chierchia, E Scola, A Falini, and ST Cappa (2014). "Neural correlates of empathic impairment in the behavioral variant of frontotemporal dementia." *Alzheimer's & Dementia* 10(6):827-834. www.ncbi.nlm.nih.gov/ pubmed/24589435. Accessed 9/10/2017.

110 Le Bouc et al.

111 Kevan.

112 The Association for Frontotemporal Degeneration, "Emotionally Absent: The Loss of Empathy and Connection in FTD." www.theaftd.org/wp-contents/ uploads/ 2014/12/PiC-fall-2014.pdf. Accessed 4/6/2016.

113 Grossman in Radin and Radin, pp 44-45.

114 Gwyneth Dickey Zakaib, "Brain Imaging Gets the Scoop on Eating Disorder in FTD." www.alzforum.org/news/research-news/brain-imaging-gets-scoop-eating-disorders-ftd. Accessed 9/10/2017.

[115] ALZFORUM, "Too Hot, Too Cold, or Just Wrong? Physiology Links Behavior to Circuits in FTD." www.alzforum.org/news/conference-coverage/too-hot-too-cold-or-just-wrong-physiology-links-behavior-circuits-ftd. Accessed 9/11/2017.

[116] Ibid.

[117] O Piguet, A Petersén, B Yin Ka Lam, S Gabery, K Murphy, JR Hodges, and GM Halliday (2011). "Eating and hypothalamus changes in behavioral-variant frontotemporal dementia." *Annals of Neurology.* 69(2):312-319. www.ncbi.nlm. nih.gov/pmc/articles/PMC3084499/. Accessed 11/23/2015.

[118] Zakaib.

[119] Rankin in Radin and Radin, p 233.

[120] The Association for Frontotemporal Degeneration, "The FTD Disorders." www.theaftd.org/understandingftd/disorders. Accessed 10/29/2016.

[121] Jonathan D Rohrer (2012), "Structural brain imaging in frontotemporal dementia." *Biochimica et Biophysica Acta* 1822:325-332. www.sciencedirect. com/ science/article/pii/S0925443911001670. Accessed 9/10/2017.

[122] Grossman in Radin and Radin, p 49.

[123] Ian G McKeith, David Burn, John O'Brien, Robert Perry, and Elaine Perry. "Chapter 91. Dementia with Lewy Bodies" in *Neuropsychopharmacology: The Fifth Generation of Progress: An Official Publication of the American College of Neuropsychopharmacology,* 5th ed. Kenneth L Davis, Dennis Charney, MD, Joseph T Coyle, and Charles Nemeroff, Md PhD (eds). (Philadelphia: Wolters Kluwer: LWW, pp 1301-1308), 2002. And Fields, p 235.

[124] S Delli Pizzi, R Franciotti, J-P Taylor, A Thomas, A Tartaro, M Onofrj, and L Bonanni (2014). "Thalamic Involvement in Fluctuating Cognition in Dementia with Lewy Bodies: Magnetic Resonance Evidences." *Cerebral Cortex* doi:10.1093/ cercor/bhu220. www.ncbi.nlm.nih.gov/ pubmed/25260701. Accessed 9/10/2017.

[125] Lewy Body Dementia Association, "Recent Studies Demonstrate Benefits of Cholinesterase Inhibitors in DLB." https://www.lbda.org/content/recent-studies-demonstrate-benefits-cholinestrase-inhibitors-dlb. Accessed 9/10/2017.

[126] Walter J Schulz-Schaeffer (2010). "The synaptic pathology of α-synuclein aggregation in dementia with Lewy bodies, Parkinson's disease and Parkinson's disease dementia." *Acta Neuropathologica.* 120(2):131-143. www.ncbi.nlm.nih. gov/pmc/articles/PMC2892607/. Accessed 11/19/15.

[127] LR Peraza, M Kaiser, M Firbank, S Graziadio, L Bonanni, M Onofrj, SJ Colloby, A Blamire, J O'Brien, and J-P Taylor (2014). "fMRI resting state networks and their association with cognitive fluctuations in dementia with Lewy bodies." *Neuroimage: Clinical* (4):558-565. www.ncbi.nlm.nih.gov/ pmc/articles/PMC 3984441/. Accessed 9/10/2017.

[128] McKeith et al.

[129] Dr. Christopher Morris, "What causes visual hallucinations in dementia with Lewy bodies?" https://www.alzheimers.org.uk/info/20053/research_ projects/679/what_causes_visual_hallucinations_in_dementia_with_lewy_ bodies. Accessed 9/10/2017.

[130] K Lobotesis, JD Fenwick, A Phipps, A Ryman, A Swann, C Ballard, IG McKeith, and JT O'Brien (2001). "Occipital hypoperfusion on SPECT in dementia with Lewy bodies but not AD." *Neurology* 56(5):643-649. www. ncbi.nlm.nih.gov/ pubmed/11245717. Accessed 11/11/2015.

[131] Peraza et al.

[132] Fields, pp 260-261.

[133] McKeith et al.

[134] Peraza et al.

[135] Whitworth and Whitworth, p 5.

Part Two

How to Be a Traveling Companion with Someone Who Has Dementia

4

The Dementia Journey

A loved one has dementia and we feel the hand of God directing us to get involved—either as a primary caregiver or as someone who comes alongside to help. Can we make a difference?

Current dementia medications may minimize the symptoms and prolong functionality, but they cannot stop the disease's progression. Additionally, loving, nurturing care has been proven to help stabilize or slow the decline. Andrew Sixsmith and his colleagues in Britain discovered some stabilization or even improvement of cognitive functions, along with slower rates of decline in loved ones, with nurturing as opposed to standard nursing home care. Sixsmith's 1993 study uncovered the essential element of humanity—the need to be loved and in community with others. These researchers called it *remitting*. This does not refer to restoring to past levels, but capitalizing on existing capabilities.[136]

In Matthew 4:4, Jesus said, "Man shall not live by bread alone, but by every word that comes from the mouth of God." People need more than physical housing; provided only with shelter, food, and water. We have a body, as well as an eternal spirit, designed to interact with others—fulfilling a plan and purpose, giving and receiving love.

Learning how to touch her soul—communicating with empathy,

showing affirming love—remains the heart of dementia care. As a close relative or friend, we can minister to her needs in a way no professional caregiver can. As her daughter, wife, or sister, we can stay by her side and remember for her.

Social interaction, activities attuned to her capabilities, and carefully structured environments, fitted to suit her current level, help preserve cognitive functions and minimize deficits. Avoiding situations where the loved one can become stressed, anxious, or fearful helps to minimize dementia symptoms. She needs environments where she feels safe and appreciated. What form this takes depends upon her unique makeup and current situation.

Acknowledging Our Denial

Our conscious mind can be slow to recognize what we understand in our heart. As I considered, once again, encouraging my mother not to shower while we were at work, I paused. A thought occurred to me— why bother; she's not going to remember. Some part of me understood my mother had cognitive issues. Another part of me dismissed it. Knowing she could be distracted and scatterbrained, I was mystified by her loss of initiative, increasing inability to organize and make decisions about her stacks of books, and her hoarding of bits of paper. I began to wonder if she was really all right at home alone. Did she need around-the-clock supervision? Then, I would shake myself back to "reality." Mom was doing fine, considering the move and the death of her husband of fifty years. It was just a phase; we would all get through it.

Denial is an ingrained coping mechanism which helps us adjust to change. Denial remains the first response to bad news. It's our instinctive defense to the fears of the unknown future. If her slide is slow and gradual, we might not come to grips with it until she is deep into the mild stages.

Discovering or acknowledging the existence of dementia often happens over a period of time as we analyze our loved ones' difficulties. Small signs add up or an event happens that forces us to realize she's not just going through a hard time; this goes beyond simple aging. Something's going on with her cognition. If she retains her verbal fluency, it's even harder to acknowledge the extent of her deficits in other areas, such as decision-making, initiative, and task completion.

Acknowledging dementia does not mean we have worked through the acceptance or accompanying grief. This is a process that takes time. It begins with the acknowledgement.

The sooner we accept the existence of dementia in our loved one, the sooner we can turn from hurt or puzzlement to concerned caregiver, remembering it's the disease, not malice, driving her behavior. This opens the door to seeking solutions that fit the reality— our loved one has a progressive degenerative disease of the brain that will alter how she perceives and reacts to the world.

Acknowledging Your Loved One's Denial

Our loved one may also experience denial. Who wants to admit the presence of dementia? Explaining away social mistakes, missed conversations, social engagements, or lost items works for a while. Reluctance to face the truth is a natural reaction. However, knowing some dementia symptoms can be caused by treatable conditions, we should encourage her to consult a doctor. See Chapter 2: Dementia Basics for more about other conditions that can produce dementia symptoms.

If your loved one is in the early stages, you might be able to help her understand. This is a hard diagnosis to accept. Come alongside, empathize, and partner with your loved one to face this foe. Dealing with denial caused by dementia will be covered in greater depth in Chapter 5: The Early-Mild Stages.

Acknowledging Grief

Even when God calls us to such a task, it doesn't mean it will be easy or that we will not feel grief, agony, or the pain of loss. We will experience the loss of companionship and fellowship we knew with our loved one. Changes will come, but God will show us the way to learn how to communicate and connect.

We grieve little-by-little with the changes—the missed vacations, hiking trips, playing tennis, and the loss of intellectual conversation and comradery. Instead of receiving encouragement and support, we now inspire, motivate, and celebrate what have now become hard-won victories. My mother used to be my confidante and my most enthusiastic supporter. That relationship melted away, but her ready smile, tender gaze, and frequent "thank-you's" remained.

God walks with us through the grief. Instead of raging at God, we rage about this disease that seems to have stolen our loved one away. We reach past our fears and cling to God's promises of sustaining grace. We search the Word of God for nuggets that will encourage us, as well as those that will strengthen us for the days ahead. We surrender our future to the God who holds us in His hands. We decide to yield to His love and not our anger. We seek to learn how to conquer evil with good and walk toward the light.

This takes time—we need to give ourselves this time to adjust to the reality of dementia in our loved one. Thankfully, we will not have to make all the changes in one day. Most diseases that cause dementia take years to run their course. Our loved one will be able to function on many levels for quite a while.

God's wisdom will help us discern what she needs today, this week, and this month. Keeping in mind that our loved one will not develop every symptom, we guard against the fear of the future. God's strength is sufficient for the day at hand—we take it one day at a time.

Accept the Caregiving Call

What if I'm not good at caregiving? Who me? God's calling me to do what? But I'm not_____. We can fill in the blank, listing all the reasons why it's not going to work. Actually, admitting that this is beyond us motivates us to seek the One who supplies the ability. Do we feel unable for the task? Are we more suited to other endeavors? This forces us to seek God's strength, and depend upon Him to enable us.

But God chose what is foolish in the world to shame the wise;
God chose what is weak in the world to shame the strong ... so
that no human being might boast in the presence of God.
1 Corinthians 1:27, 29

The God who created the universe in an instant is able to supply our needs. Do we not trust Him? He promises to help in our time of need (Hebrews 4:16). We can take every hopeless situation and exhausting night to Him. He will provide, supply, and sustain. We do not walk this path alone if we are a child of God, indwelt by the Holy Spirit, and with the Son of God interceding for us.

It is an honor and a privilege to be called of God to minister to others. The calling to help our loved one finish well is a vital mission as important as helping the neighbor next door or those dwelling in distant lands. There are secret blessings to serving others. When we share God's love with the help of the Holy Spirit, His love flows through us (Romans 5:5). It enriches and sustains us as we minister the love of God to others.

If Christ could endure the cross for us, we can, with His help, endure the years of helping our loved ones with dementia. Whenever I felt a little pity party beginning, I remembered my sacrifice was much less than Christ's. In John 15:12, Christ commanded us to love one another. "This is my commandment, that you love one another as I have loved you." How could I not help my mother through her final journey?

To Honor Your Spouse

"But from the beginning of creation, 'God made them male
and female." Therefore a man shall leave his father and
mother and hold fast to his wife, and the two shall become

*one flesh.' So they are no longer two but one flesh. What
therefore God has joined together, let not man separate."*
Mark 10:6-9

Neither must dementia separate a man from his wife or a woman
from her husband. If God led a couple together in marriage, He
can lead them together through the valley of dementia. If one has
dementia, God can guide the other in the caregiving task.

The husband of a friend of mine developed Lewy body dementia.
She said, "I know that God has a reason for this and it doesn't matter
that I don't understand why He has allowed this, but it does matter
that I depend on Him to show me how to proceed on this journey.
I find myself amazed at how I respond most of the time to … [my
husband's] mistakes or bathroom messes. He thinks he is doing things
right and he is not. It indeed is mentally draining, but that's okay. I
only hope and pray that I can help him finish well. It is also amazing
to me, how God has prepared me to be his helper at this time."[137]
    She went on to describe how the Lord led her to take care of her
mother-in-law when her children were teenagers; look after an aging
neighbor; and be a good friend to many of the older ladies in her
church. Her heart's burden to help, exercised by caring for others in
the past, equipped her for her calling and ministry to her husband.

Dr. Robertson McQuilkin, an internationally known professor of
biblical ethics, resigned as president of Columbia Bible College and
Seminary to care for Muriel, his wife. She was diagnosed with early
onset Alzheimer's at age 58. Although to some people this would
seem to be a hopeless situation, Dr. McQuilkin found the liberty
Christ spoke about in Luke 17:33, "Whoever seeks to preserve his life
will lose it, but whoever loses his life will keep it."[138]

While caring for his wife with her bathroom accidents, times of wandering, and irrational behaviors, he discovered a deeper love for his wife and God. He realized, "It's the nearest thing I've experienced on a human plane to what my relationship with God was designed to be: God's unfailing love poured out in constant care of helpless me."[139]

Sometimes, we feel tempted to give in to self-love, which is an ever-narrowing search to fulfill our own pleasures. Our wants and desires become ensnaring obsessions and lusts. God created us as servants—we find our greatest joy reaching beyond ourselves to help others. The constraints and difficulties of caring for our loved one become our gateway to closer intimacy with God and His love. As He enables us to sacrificially minister to our loved one, we begin to experience God's blossoming in our life.

That our "bondage" to caregiving is our gateway to growing in Christ, that our shackles of caring for someone dependent upon us brings freedom, and that our fears of the sorrows of the dementia valley instead become our garden of joy seems to be beyond all understanding.[140] The Apostle Paul stated in Philippians 4:4-7 that in the midst of hard times, by clinging to God in prayer with thanksgiving, we can have "the peace of God, which surpasses all understanding."

Dr. McQuilkin considered it a "high honor" to be called of God to minister to his wife.[141] I, too, felt the blessings of caring for my mother. I always felt privileged, along with my sisters, to have been chosen to help her.

Muriel had Alzheimer's disease and retained her ability to feel emotions and respond, even if she did not fully understand. However, with frontotemporal types of dementia, the ability to perceive others' emotions and respond with feeling is often impaired in the early stages. Called *emotional blunting,* the loved one can become emotively unresponsive, making it feel like your spouse has been transformed into a stranger.[142]

When the ability to respond seeps away, choosing to love her is more important than ever. Even if she cannot react the way she used to, her essential being has not departed. She is still the person you married; she has not disappeared, even though her reactions have altered. How does one cope with such changes in someone close to us?

Taking a more distant, objective approach helps. Caregivers who can see themselves as caregivers instead of family have greater peace and success.[143] Being able to mentally shift to caregiver enables us to put aside our emotional attachments, past history, hopes, and fears.

To Honor Your Parent

"Honor your father and mother" (this is the first commandment with a promise), "that it may go well with you and that you may live long in the land."
Ephesians 6:2-3

How do we honor our parents when dementia enters the family? The goal is to see our loved one has the optimal, loving, nurturing care and safest environment we can find with the available resources. We need to look to her heartfelt needs. We need not fear or resist participating since God will work his ways through our lives while we shoulder the burdens for this calling.

It's a commitment to seek what's best for her (which might not always feel good at the time). The answers will vary from family to family, as well as from month to month. Yes, in some cases, temporarily making changes to care for her in her home is the right thing to do, however the "right answer" might change as her dementia progresses. For other families, the Lord leads in different directions. Whether just the right assisted living facility, skilled nursing home, adult day care, or home health care services, God can and does work through all these options.

If both parents are alive, we become part of the supportive network for the one dealing with a spouse with dementia. We can advise, suggest, and aid, but the primary caregiving falls on the parent without dementia. If choices made do not work well, we continue to encourage, provide support, and pray.

Look for God's Help

For no one can lay a foundation other than that which is laid, which is Jesus Christ.
1 Corinthians 3:11

Tasks that seem beyond our capacities are possible with God. He is our all in all, our sure foundation, and the inner life force which sees us through each day. The wisdom to see unique solutions comes from God—"the fear of the Lord is the beginning of wisdom" (Proverbs 1:7). How do we figure out a way to connect with our loved one as her world rotates away from us? Where do the ideas come from that solve nagging problems? They come from God.

In many ways, God will direct and guide us. He can work through the advice of our medical team, other caregivers, staff, care group friends, books, and the internet, as well as through prayer and journaling.

If we have been leaning on others for spiritual strength instead of the Lord, this is the time to put aside crutches and live each day abiding in Him (John 15:4-5). "I can do all things through him who strengthens me" (Philippians 4:13). If God is the center and strength of our life, we can persevere and help our loved one through her valley. He can transform us into the loving caregiver we long to be.

This physical life is the prelude to our heavenly future. This life, with all its trials and tribulations, is our earthly boot camp, preparing us for heaven. This is also our loved ones' challenge to face, as well. Would we even consider abandoning her to walk this valley alone? May it never be.

Sidebar: The "Why" Question

We naturally ask "Why?" when bad things happen. We seek to find the reason God allowed our loved one to develop dementia. Job's friends asked him what sin brought disaster upon him (Job 22:4-5).

Hebrews 12 teaches that God disciplines His children (Hebrews 12:3-13). This is not punishment, but correction. While God can allow bad things in our lives to force us to deal with unconfessed sin, we cannot assume that the existence of dementia points to error in a person's life. Rather, the emergence of cognitive loss can be the means God will use to bring glory to Himself. Others will see the love and grace of God in the testimony of the patient endurance of the loved one and our caregiving (John 13:34-35).

God works through hard times. He can turn bad into good as we walk with Him through the valley of suffering. A sovereign God determines our lifespan, as well as the diseases that will deliver us from this mortal world to the next (Ecclesiastes 3:1-4).

Why dementia? If not dementia, by what other means would I choose for my mother to graduate to heaven? Only God knows the end from the beginning (Isaiah 46:10). Only God can see the glory in the midst of sorrow. Only by trusting God and choosing to walk with Him can we begin to find our way through it.

For now, on this side of eternity, we don't need to know the answer, just the way. Truly, Jesus stated He is the way, the truth, and the life (John 14:6). He is the answer to our whys.

Look for a Support Network

Being called as the primary caregiver for a loved one with dementia does not mean you have to do it all yourself. Eventually, the loved one will be completely dependent on others. No one can provide total care for another by themselves.

The most successful caregivers utilize a variety of helpers and services. Many can tap into family for help taking care of the house, lawn, or with finances. Close friends might take the loved one to appointments, or for short excursions. Depending upon the loved one's capabilities, adult daycare might work for a few days each week. Many facilities offer respite programs where someone can stay for short periods of time. See Chapter 6 The Middle-Moderate Stages for dealing with the caregiving burden and burnout. As caregivers, we need to maintain an objective viewpoint of our loved one's changing needs as she progresses, keeping our limitations in mind.

The Caregiving Goal

And one of them, a lawyer, asked him a question to test him.
"Teacher, which is the great commandment in the Law?"
And he said to him, "You shall love the Lord your God with
all your heart and with all your soul and with all your mind.
This is the great and first commandment. And a second is
like it: You shall love your neighbor as yourself. On these two
commandments depend all the Law and the Prophets."
Matthew 22:35-40

The main goal is to help our loved one live well with dementia for the full amount of time God has given her.

Love dictates the path by which we advance. This is a committed love that seeks the best for your loved one, even if she becomes angry in the short-term. We teach ourselves to respond with love and patience, not returning harsh words with angry outbursts. We follow Christ's example who gave up His life that we might live.

For our sake he made him to be sin who knew no sin,
so that in him we might become the righteousness of God.
2 Corinthians 5:21

This type of love seeks the best for the loved one—it's not mushy, squishy, or saccharine. If she has reached the point where she no longer understands the consequences of her actions, we must step in and make the decision—it's time to give up the car, or you can no longer live on your own. Loving does not mean allowing her to continue activities that would now be harmful, such as driving or cooking on her own. Exercising love is not always easy as we seek ways to honor and respect her as an image-bearer of God in the midst of her growing dependency.

My mother could rotate instantly from sage-like wisdom to a childlike dependency, looking to me for help with aching feet or a sore throat.

While on a shopping trip for items for her new place at Sienna Crest, I remarked I needed a new purse. She encouraged me to go to the purse section in the department store. I was not optimistic. A purse I had purchased from this store had worn out within a year.

As we arrived at the section she looked over, pointed to a purse and said, "That one."

Running through scenarios on how to politely disagree, I looked over, prepared to dismiss the choice. Then, I took a closer look, examined the strap connections and number of pockets. Incredibly, amazingly, Mom had picked out just the perfect purse, which lasted for many years.

Sharon, an aide at Sienna Crest, always told us as we visited our loved ones to never forget they still knew many things and had a lot to share. As I carried my purse, it reminded me to always be on the lookout for Mom's gems of wisdom.

The Value of Our Loved One

Is my humanity based on my intelligence, how far I can run, or whether I can paint a portrait or write a song? Of course not. As our capabilities wax and wane throughout our lives, our essential humanness never leaves. All people are created in the image of God (Genesis 1:26). Whether brilliant or average, athletically gifted, or musically inclined, with all our variable traits and personalities, we remain human, even in the midst of disability.

Our loved one did not cease to be human when the dementia appeared. Yes, some of her capacities have changed; how she perceives the world has been altered, but her humanity remains. Even if she cannot do all the things she used to do, she can still love God and fulfill His purpose for her. No disease, not even Alzheimer's, can erase the image of God in a person.

If we lose our mind and memories, what remains? What of our relationship to God and those we love? Does the body become an empty shell? Has our humanity left? People fear dementia above most other diseases.[144]

Our value does not lie in our memories of our past or our community, nor in our physical abilities. Since we are created in God's image and He put a high value on us, we find our worth in God. We are spiritual as well as physical beings. Even if our organic brain is impaired, the value of our life remains.

People with dementia are very much alive. We must never forget to search for ways to enable our loved ones to interact with others, and to give and receive love. We can find ways to respect her humanity according to her present capabilities.

Next Steps:

Extending the Offer to Be the Caregiver

Being willing and extending an offer to help might not always be met with gratitude and a smile. My mother graciously let me help with various activities as I saw her struggling. Many individuals, fearing loss of control or feeling anxiety about letting anyone help, might not accept your offer nor respond with thankfulness.

Help as much as she will let you, but if she decides to go a different way, let her go, keeping the door of communication open. She might prefer another family member or be ready to accept your help later. At least you extended the offer.

Sometimes, we can only pray if she shuts us out of her life in the belief that we are cheating her or stealing from her. As much as it depends upon us, we must strive to live peaceably with all men, even those who think the worst of us (Romans 12:18).

Remember, the extent of her ambivalence against you may be the result of the disease. Her disorientation, confusion, fear, and the effects of anosognosia (see chapters 3 and 5 for more discussion on this topic) might convince your loved one you are the enemy. Despite the deep hurt we feel when accused of wrongdoing, try not to let the accusations or behavior build a wall between you. Give the hurts to the Lord.

If your loved one feels more comfortable with another family member helping with finances and other matters, that's fine. As long as the family can come together to support the loved one, you have achieved your goal. Perhaps God is calling us to be a friend who can visit her, or to take her places when her primary caregiver cannot (the primary caregiver will also need help).

If she becomes suspicious of us, we might have to let her go. But, never forget to pray for her. We can do everything we can to stay in touch and available if our loved one changes her mind. One woman waited until her mother with dementia was ready to accept her help. Although it was a difficult period when her mother directed her anger toward her, the daughter's perseverance bore fruit. In time, her mother asked for her help.[145]

What If No One Else in the Family Will Help?

There is often one primary caregiver. Availability might lead other family members (who might live just as close to the loved one) to leave the burden to one individual.

We must resist letting a root of bitterness infect us. "See to it that no one fails to obtain the grace of God; that no 'root of bitterness' springs up and causes trouble, and by it many become defiled" (Hebrews 12:15). Bitterness hurts us as well as those around us, and poisons our souls. If the Lord called us to help our loved ones and other family members do not pitch in to help, they will be the ones losing out on the blessings. We can only control ourselves. We can determine to forgive and to move on with caring for our loved one.

Forcing other family members to help can be counterproductive. Whatever their reasons—fear of commitment, feeling life is already too busy, or the inability to accept the changes in their loved one— committing them in prayer to God and moving on is our best option. Perhaps when we stop pushing them to help, they might freely choose to join us.[146]

What If the Family Is Divided?

Dementia can sneak up on a family. Those closest to the loved one might realize she has dementia, but other family members who live far away and only talk briefly with her on the phone might not have accepted this fact. If she has anosognosia, she might also be creating confabulations—stories that correlate with her version of reality (see chapter 3). This can fracture the family with one side trying to help her live with dementia while the other side accuses them of ganging up on her.

Some families deal with this by encouraging those who are in denial spend a significant amount of time with the loved one. Hopefully as they observe her behavior over longer periods, they will see that while she can chat for an hour on the phone, she does struggle with her thinking. Only after spending time with her will the reality become evident.[147]

While this phase can cause distress as she and the family might resist necessary changes, we persist until everyone eventually accepts the solutions and put them into place. This takes time and can be a progressive, step-by-step effort. In the beginning, the family could use organizations like Meals on Wheels and employ home health aides. These options may suffice until the time to move or find living arrangements with around-the-clock care.

Rotate to a Caregiver Mindset

The reality of dementia in a family brings change. How our loved one acts will change; her ability to function and care for herself will diminish over time; and what we need to be for her will also change.

We remain her husband or daughter or son, but if needed, we also become her primary caregiver. This sometimes requires a conscious awareness of stepping out of one role and into another. We agree to be her comforter, confidante, advocate, caregiver, and administrator. We will probably have to make some difficult decisions for our loved one as her ability to think and reason degrades.

If our spouse develops dementia, we have to relinquish his former role and service to us, understanding the way he expresses his love will change. Yes, there will be times we can interact as husband and wife (and this can happen with the Lewy body dementia diseases). Other times, we will act as care provider. As we begin to shoulder more and more responsibility with his growing dependency, we always strive to honor his humanity.

When our loved ones do change, it is not out of spite, trying to get even, or a conscious decision to stop loving others. The brain's ability to monitor and control reactions, or to generate emotional warmth, is under attack. It's not a choice, but an outworking of damaged brain networks that no longer function as in the past. We have to remember to blame the disease and not give into thinking he no longer loves us, doesn't care, or is deliberately trying to hurt us.

We built emotional ties with our loved one. Our lives have been intertwined. We must let go of the ways he used to be with us. If our spouse was the family's financial wizard and we are useless when it comes to money, finding a trustworthy son or daughter can fill the gap. While our emotional bonds with our spouse or parent will change, our relationships are not over, just different.

Instead of my mother being my ardent supporter, I became hers. As we let go of how the relationship used to be, we begin to accept the new dynamic. We continue to show her every respect as we take on responsibilities she can no longer shoulder. We seek to find the *new normal*, looking for new joys and blessings. Some children have reestablished close relationships that had been fractured in the past.

Dr. John Zeisel, a designer of dementia units for nursing homes, recommends keeping a log of our loved one's likes and preferences and his reactions, discovering the warp and woof of his emerging personality.[148] Even with the changes, he will always be your dad or husband. His essential personhood and individuality remains even though the way he is with us in the present has changed.

The physiological changes in our loved one will result in what appears to be a different person. He, as an individual, remains, even though he now acts differently. His food preferences might have changed if he is struggling with frontotemporal dementia. He may now wish to avoid noisy museums or the busyness of local fairs or markets. Yet, he is still your loved one. You can unearth the secrets of his new personality and ways of being. You can study and adjust how you interact to give and receive love. It will have a different tempo and might involve different props and backgrounds, but you can still connect in love.

Become Your Loved One's Advocate

Seeing ourselves as executive director, we seek the best possible care for our loved one, marshaling available resources to provide the best solutions for our loved one's current stage; knowing the answers will change with the disease's progression. Our goal is to seek the best for our loved one, whether it feels good at the moment or not; whether it matches our plans or not.

We might not necessarily be the best one for daily care, or we might be. We need to set aside our desire to do everything for our loved one and gather the best care resources. We can oversee them and make sure they follow through. Since each person is unique, the optimal living arrangement will vary from individual to individual, and from stage to stage. My mother was an outgoing gregarious person who came alive in the company of others. She loved Sienna Crest for its open community. She would not have done as well isolated at home with full-time home health aides. Other individuals may do better at home.

While our first instinct might be to jump in and take over, if we are not the first-line caregiver—for example, our mother might be the caregiver for our father with dementia—we might not be in a position to make all the decisions. Sometimes, God calls us to come alongside and support the primary caregiver.

Habilitate vs. Rehabilitate

Good dementia care seeks to optimize the loved one's capabilities. A group of caregivers in the 1990s called this *habilitation*. This is different from the standard recovery model for rehabilitation care, which seeks to return the loved one to full recovery. For example, rehabilitation will try to orient the loved one to the world, while habilitation will seek to help the loved one orient to the world as she sees it.

Habilitation therapy looks at the whole person—health, speech, cognition, as well as her environment—and strives to stabilize current capabilities. Treating everything, this therapy model focuses on stimulating remaining functionality, physical as well as mental. We meet her in her world, allowing her to be as independent as possible, only limited by safety considerations.

Treatments range from standard medications, structured therapies and activities, as well as altering the environment to optimize our loved one's competencies. Seeking to maximize abilities, the goal is to help maintain a positive mood throughout the day. It heads off trouble before it starts and simplifies caregiving.[149]

For example, ongoing care would include ensuring pain from arthritis or other ailments is properly treated, thus reducing outbursts due to pain. If she can no longer remember to take her pain medication, caregivers can administer it to her instead. Even if she can no longer verbalize her hunger or other distresses, we need to discern her needs and help her remain calm.

We can structure the physical layout of the home to help overcome apathy, to remove obstacles, and to encourage participation. Accommodations can include setting out fewer choices, removing clutter, using contrasting colors on the floors and walls, enhancing the lighting, and modifying the rooms to help her navigate her surroundings throughout the day.

We can develop social activities to help her successfully connect with others through *failure-free* activities that provide a sense of acceptance and accomplishment. This includes not challenging our loved ones in areas where she has cognitive losses, and limiting her exposure to environments and social situations which create confusion.[150] Based upon her favorite interests, music, food and activities, her daily routines help her to stay positive throughout the day.

We Enable Our Loved Ones to Do as Much as Possible

By focusing on what she can do instead of what she lost, we help her stay actively involved, only providing help as needed. For example, if she has trouble deciding what to eat for breakfast, we can set out a few options she can choose from instead of pointing her to the pantry. We might have to put the toothpaste on the toothbrush and help her get started brushing. As she moves through the various stages, we will need to pay attention to areas where greater accommodation is required.

Since she can have good days, we need to let her try to do as much as possible. Some days, she can do most of an activity on her own, while she might need more assistance the next day. Staying alert, we respond to her present needs.

It is easy to take over and do everything for her. This not only will accelerate her decline—if she doesn't use it, she will lose it more quickly—it also does not respect her. We all need to feel useful and capable. Letting her do what she can, will help her feel whole. It might take longer, it might be messier or not be up to the standard she used to have, but she will accomplish something.

With varying abilities, particularly with Lewy body dementia, what she can do safely on her own might fluctuate greatly. So, try it out. If she can't do it that day, no problem, we pick up the slack. If she can do it that day—the neurons connect, she remembers, and gets it done—that's a wonderful day to remember! We can watch for overcoming obstacles that keep her from participating. Does she need help getting started, can we make it easier or simpler, or can she participate at a lower level?

Eventually, her abilities will diminish or seem to disappear in an ebb and flow of good days and bad days. Expect change. It will keep us flexible and on the lookout for signs that she progressed to the next level.

Enjoy what you can with your loved one, get out, have adventures, go places, do things for as long as possible. The upside to the progression is some problem behaviors may also diminish. My mom, with the family gene for worry, eventually progressed to the point that she forgot to worry—a blessing in disguise. As long as she could handle it, we took her to the zoo with the grandkids, walked the mall, went shopping and out to dinner. She even traveled to Colorado for a wedding before her world shrank and we had to take the sweet treats and adventures to her.

Stages

Early-Mild Stage ⚬⚬ Late Autumn

The loved one is still capable in many areas. Enable her to stay active, but provide more help as deficits increase. Make plans for the future.

Middle-Moderate Stages ⚬⚬ Early Winter

Ensure the loved one is safe, nurtured, and cared for. Try to keep her engaged to the fullest extent. Outings will be closer to home.

Late-Severe Stages ৯৫ Hard Winter

The loved one reaches total dependency. Her world shrinks as earthly interests fall away. Rotate to comfort care as the end draws near.

The dementia pathway has been broken down into stages based on our loved one's cognitive levels and abilities. The stages vary from four or more, and differ greatly from disease to disease. The major disease types highlighted in this book—Alzheimer's disease, vascular cognitive impairment, frontotemporal dementia, and Lewy body dementia—are broad categories for many different diseases with their own unique progression. For example, the exact symptoms differ greatly, depending upon where the disease starts with frontotemporal dementia. But, overall, our loved one will have greater difficulties as the disease process develops.

It is beyond the scope of this book to detail the staging sequences for the various diseases. However, overall disease progression typically follows a three-step staging model: *early-mild, middle-moderate,* and *late-severe.* Each step encompasses two or more stages in the disease process. For this reason, we will refer to these stages in the plural.

The progression through the stages does not occur in a linear fashion, but moves back and forth, sometimes missing, and then usually missing, until the ability disappears altogether (we think).[51] Some days, the remaining neurons connect and she communicates better than she has in weeks. There will be times of the day when our loved one will be at her peak. Some days, everyone will struggle—the caregivers and the loved one. Dementia affects us all—we can commiserate together.

Understanding the stage your loved one presently inhabits helps in discerning her current capabilities, strengths, and weaknesses. Staging provides benchmarks for selecting appropriate therapies. We can help her stay engaged if we willingly adjust daily activities to current levels. Eventually, the loved one will slide into greater dependency as she progresses to the middle stages with moderate symptoms, usually requiring more care. The decline accelerates as the deficits compound until death approaches in the late stages. The speed of progression and the exact nature of the deficits may vary, but the trajectory continues—greater disability over time until death approaches.

Each stage brings its own challenges, heartaches, and blessings. Treasure the time with your loved one: enjoy the fun parts, find the solutions to the difficulties, and pray through obstacles and looming mountains. With God all things are possible, even reaching out in love to your loved one.

Early–Mild Stages

Beginning early in the disease, the symptoms are mild and the family is just becoming aware of the problem. When we come alongside as her caregiver, we investigate, plan, and lay ahead for the future. As we enable her to do as much as possible, we gradually take on responsibilities when she can no longer manage them.

Middle–Moderate Stages

During the middle-moderate stages, we should shoulder many of the burdens of life such as paying bills, working with financial advisers, or arranging home maintenance. This will free him up to enjoy the sunrise and watch a flock of turkeys meander their way across the field, or the hummingbird drink from tiger lily flowers. As the mounting deficits seem to change our loved one, we strive to adapt to his *new normal*. This is the time to ensure he is safe and secure, while enabling him to participate in life.

Late–Severe Stages

In the late-severe stages, our loved one will be severely incapacitated, struggling to move, see, hear, and know. We still need to enable them to do as much as possible with evolving accommodations to match advancing deficits.

At the end, our loved one will be bedridden. We need to understand how and when to rotate toward comfort care. We support our loved one as his days draw to a close.

Great variety exists between the symptoms appearing in the early and middle stages. However as our loved ones' dementia advances with the disease(s) and more areas of the brain are compromised, the differences lessen. Toward the end, most dementia sufferers will have some problems with memory, behaviors, speech, and movement. Jan Zimmerman, a nursing administrator for Heritage Homes in Watertown, Wisconsin, said that the greatest challenge with anyone struggling with dementia is the communication issue. "As far as the decline in functionality with things, it's pretty consistent across the board with them."[152]

Not Everyone Goes through Every Stage

Not everyone with dementia progresses through the final stages. Some will die of other diseases or complications, such as pneumonia, before the brain loses its ability to keep the body alive.[153] Hospice is a great resource and help if our loved one does progress to the end stages of dementia.

The Joys and Sorrows of the Dementia Journey

The Sacrifice of Praise

For here we have no lasting city, but we seek the city that is to come. Through him then let us continually offer up a sacrifice of praise to God, that is, the fruit of lips that acknowledge his name.
Hebrews 13:14-15

"The heavy heart lifts on the wings of praise."[154] In the midst of the sorrows, heartaches, and difficulties, we can praise God. This includes thanksgiving. In 1 Thessalonians 5:18, we find the command to " …give thanks in all circumstances; for this is the will of God in Christ Jesus for you." In our praise, we surrender to the will of God, releasing anger, bitterness, and resentment.

Even with the changes dementia brings, we can still experience life in all its vibrancy and wonder. We keep our eyes on Christ, striving to keep the 30,000-foot view. We can still laugh at the funny moments—ours as well as those we love. As we reorder our priorities, we re-examine what's most important—loving God and others. We are just passing through this earth to a glorious heavenly future. We endure, knowing better times will be ours in the end.

Judy Towne Jennings' husband developed Lewy body dementia. As a physical therapist, she understood how life-changing this diagnosis would be. In her book, *Living with Lewy Body Dementia*, she shares the lessons she learned while helping her husband live with this disease. Judy said, "When faced with major life decisions that are difficult, require hard work, and offer no guarantee of success, I offer this suggestion: assume an adventure attitude."[155] They went on three cruises, Judy found ways to help her husband play tennis as long as possible, and they joked and teased each other, striving not to miss the day's humor. She helped him stay active while she encouraged herself to rise to the occasion, even when taking on tasks she had never done before. She added, "Pessimism is easy, optimism takes work … With positive thinking, there is a greater chance that the inevitable anger, rage, and frustrations will be manageable."[156]

When my mother forgot words, or lost her train of thought, she laughed. If the doctor asked her questions she couldn't answer, she laughed. Laughter is a safety valve.

A glad heart makes a cheerful face,
but by sorrow of heart the spirit is crushed.
Proverbs 15:13

Shortly after my firstborn son died of sudden infant death syndrome, I asked the Lord why this happened. A question arose in my mind. What would my choice have been: having Jonathan for four-and-a-half months or never knowing him at all? Instantly, I knew I would take whatever time God granted me with my firstborn son. Let us not waste the time God provides to us with our loved ones.

When considering the sacrifices involved in helping our loved ones with dementia finish well, we also must consider the treasured time afforded us. Yes, it will be difficult, and hard to watch. Some months, it seemed to go on and on with no end in sight. Yet, would I have traded those six years helping my Mom for having more free time? Never; no way! So, we can step up to the plate, accept the challenge, decide in our hearts to care for our loved one as we would want our loved one to care for us, and help her finish well.

---

[136] Andrew Sixsmith, John Stilwell, and John Copeland (1993). "'Rementia': Challenging the limits of Dementia Care," *International Journal of Geriatric Psychiatry* 8(12): 993-1000. https://eurekamag.com/pdf.php?pdf=008011198. Accessed 9/15/2017.

[137] Received February 2, 2016 in an email from my friend Bonnie.

[138] Robertson McQuilkin, *A Promise Kept* (Carol Stream, IL: Tyndale House Publishers, Inc., 2006), p 35.

[139] Ibid., p 33.

[140] Pages 32-36 in Dr. McQuilkin's book, *A Promise Kept*, expound on the deeper love we experience as we exercise sacrificial love, versus the devastating outcomes from refusing to love unconditionally in a marriage.

[141] Ibid., p 23.

[142] Rankin in Radin and Radin, p 238.

[143] KW Hepburn, J Tornatore, B Center, and SW Ostwald, "Dementia Family Caregiver Training: Affecting Beliefs about Caregiving and Caregiver Outcomes," *Journal of the American Geriatrics* Society 49(2001): 450-457 cited by Rankin in Radin and Radin, p 239.

[144] John Swinton, *Dementia: Living in the Memories of God* (Grand Rapids, MI: William B Eerdmans Publishing Company, 2012), p 187.

[145] Jade C Angelica, *Where Two Worlds Touch: A Spiritual Journey through Alzheimer's Disease* (Boston: Skinner House Books, 2014), p 119.

[146] Evelyn McLay and Ellen P Young, *Mom's OK, She Just Forgets: The Alzheimer's Journey from Denial to Acceptance* (Amherst, NY: Prometheus Books, 2006), p 72.

[147] Ibid., p 57.

[148] Zeisel, pp 183-184.

[149] Paul Raia, PhD, "Chapter 2 Habilitation Therapy: A New Starscape." https://www.nhqualitycampaign.org/files/Habilitation_Therapy_a_New_starscape2.edit.pdf. Accessed 6/17/2016.

[150] Ibid.

[151] Cummings, p 219.

[152] Jan Zimmerman, RN, Nursing Administrator, Heritage Homes, Watertown, WI. Interview 5/20/2014.

[153] Nancy L Mace, MA, and Peter V Rabins, MD, MPH, *The 36-Hour Day: A Family Guide to Caring for People Who Have Alzheimer's Disease, Related Dementias, and Memory Loss*, 5th ed. (New York: Grand Central Life & Style, 2012), p 203.

[154] McQuilkin, p 62.

[155] Judy Towne Jennings PT, MA, *Living with Lewy Body Dementia: One Caregiver's Personal, In-Depth Experience* (Bloomington, IN: WestBow Press, a Division of Thomas Nelson, 2012), p 12.

[156] Ibid., p 13 for quote; see also pages 20-28, 35 for descriptions of their daily adventures.

5

The Early-Mild Stages

For everything there is a season, and a time
for every matter under heaven:
Ecclesiastes 3:1

E ach stage is a transition with its own unique joys, obstacles, and troubles. The early-mild stages, transitioning from independence to dependence, mark the beginning of the changes to our loved one's life. Adjustments, such as where he lives or works, will need to be made as disability increases. Dementia means our loved one's cognitive problems have begun to impact his ability to handle daily affairs: manage schedules and appointments, pay bills and control spending, respond appropriately to co-workers and family, communicate fluently, or complete projects.

While our loved one can remain active, socially engaged, and involved, the ways and means will change. Along the way, we will care, guide, and direct as new solutions to our loved one's needs become necessary, one by one.

This in-between time, when our loved one can still maintain a level of independence but his capabilities are melting away, carries risks. How long can he safely live on his own, manage his finances, or continue driving? How can we help him transition to a safe place where he can progress through the latter stages? Should he move in with us (can our homes and lifestyles accommodate this), or move to an appropriate facility? Or, can he continue to live on his own for a while?

Pat Summitt, the former head woman's basketball coach at Tennessee University, was not only diagnosed with early-onset Alzheimer's disease, as the public person she was, she also did not try to hide it. Instead, she announced her diagnosis. She explained that people in the earlier stages of dementia were still capable individuals, able to reason and act.[157] She continued to be active for as long as possible. Diagnosed with early-onset Alzheimer's at the age of 59, Pat Summitt passed away at 64. She continued to inspire by serving as coach emeritus after her diagnosis.

Push for Correct Diagnosis

To go forward, be persistent in getting a diagnosis that makes sense with the symptoms you see in your loved one. Sometimes, it takes several attempts before the correct disease has been identified. Lewy body and the frontotemporal dementias might be misdiagnosed as depression, anxiety, menopause, bipolar, Alzheimer's disease, or Parkinson's disease.

Sidebar: Early-Mild Common Characteristics

Alzheimer's disease (AD)- Vascular cognitive impairment (VCI)

Mild decline with memory problems; repeats questions, stories, or actions; gets lost in familiar areas; often misplaces items and may start accusing others of taking items; has increased trouble planning, doing math, analyzing, and problem-solving; decreased activity levels, with loss of initiative. While AD usually has a more consistent downhill trend, VCI often follows a pathway similar to AD in a steplike manner. See chapter 3 for greater detail.

Frontotemporal dementia (FTD)

Depending on the lobe where the damage begins, might start with strange behaviors and abrupt personality shifts, loss of speech fluency, or loss of the ability to empathize and understand others' feelings.

Lewy body dementia (LBD)

Periods of confusion; REM sleep behavior disorder (RBD); hallucinations; beginning to have problems starting or completing tasks; impaired reasoning, but memory usually not affected in the beginning; and might have problems with movement.

Considerations for the Early-Mild Stages

While the deficits are just beginning and mostly mild, they will still interfere with our loved one's ability to function. Many abilities will remain untouched at this point. The trick is discerning where and when to offer needed help—we should not attempt to do everything for our loved one, even if she can't complete the action as she did in the past. Everyone needs to adjust to our loved one's *new normal*.

Changes will occur, usually slowly, but can also accelerate at times. Onset of other medical concerns, such as infections or accidents, can send our loved one spiraling down. Medications and surgery can cause our loved one's cognition to deteriorate. She might eventually stabilize, but never quite regain her former capabilities.

While she retains her maturity, she may seem like a seven-year-old in certain areas—such as needing help with common ailments such as a sore throat. She may be able to still lecture in her field of expertise, but might need help with scheduling or getting to the venue. With her uneven abilities, we need to extend help when and where it's needed. Not all capabilities disappear in the early stages. In some ways, she can still counsel and advise us. In other ways, she needs us to take care of her.

We need to be alert to her growing need for more care, help, or advice while continuing to show her every respect and courtesy. This drives us to look to God to supply the wisdom to traverse this path. On her good days, my mother would respond with her old wit and wisdom. Some days, the brain connected enough of the pieces to think and communicate.

The ability to perceive others' emotions often remains with Alzheimer's-type dementia. Our loved one may pick up on the emotions we project, even though she may not be able to explain it. Are we not really listening? Are we impatient? Are we trying to force the situation or manipulate them? We need to be calm, patient, and present with her; we need to control our own emotions, paying attention to how we react to her. The ability to perceive other's emotions might be impaired to some extent with frontotemporal dementias.

Her body language will speak to us, as well. We need to not only listen to the words, but also the underlying emotions. Does she appear stressed, bewildered, or frustrated? Does she sit quietly in a corner during family gatherings while she used to participate freely? The sooner we tune in to where she is, the sooner we will begin to comprehend her needs.

Get It in Writing

Legal Documents—The time to help her draw up various powers of attorney and an advance directive detailing her end of life care decisions is when she can articulate her choices for future decisions. These are difficult discussions, but one of the gifts of getting an early diagnosis is having the time to help your loved one state her preferences in writing. Find a good attorney knowledgeable about the state's laws to help your loved one draw up the necessary documents.

Too many families delay these discussions, thinking they could deal with these issues at a more opportune time, only to find that something has rendered the loved one no longer able to vocalize her wishes. Disease progression can range from a few years to more than ten. Even if you think your loved one will sail along for a while in the mild stages, discussing end-of-life issues sooner rather than later is wise. An unexpected infection, accident, or surgical procedure could quickly push her past the point where she can articulate her choices.

Mom and I visited a local attorney who specialized in eldercare. She helped Mom complete legal documents, such as financial and health care powers of attorney, discussing options with her such as whether she wanted to be resuscitated or would agree to a feeding tube.

⸺✦XX✦X✦XX✦✦⸺

Sidebar: Differences between Advance Directives, Living Wills, and Durable Powers of Attorney for Health Care

Each state has its own laws and regulations concerning advance directives, living wills, and durable powers of attorney for health care. Usually, an advance directive or living will states what level of medical care and treatment your loved one would like in the event of an injury, illness, or accident; while the durable power of attorney for health care designates a representative to make medical decisions when your loved one becomes incapacitated.

Some states fold the living will into an advance directive; others consider the living will and durable power of attorney for health care an advance directive. The common thread is the opportunity to put choices concerning treatment options, such as use of ventilators, cardiopulmonary resuscitation, or tube feeding in writing. The doctor(s) will interpret the advance directive to guide current medical treatment. In some states, the choices of the living will are incorporated into the power of attorney form.

A durable power of attorney for health care selects a designated representative to enforce your loved one's preferences. It allows your loved one to pick a trusted representative to speak for her when she can no longer speak for herself. The caregiver has the authority to request treatment. Instead of a doctor trying to decipher your loved one's wishes, the trusted representative can react to current circumstances.

Joni Eareckson Tada, president and CEO of Joni & Friends, an international disability advocacy group, is familiar with the necessity of choosing the right person to speak on someone's behalf. She has lived most of her adult life as a quadriplegic. She stated that a representative with personal knowledge of the individual is a better advocate than relying on a piece of paper.[158] She explained that some medical professionals believe people who have completed living wills do not want medical interventions. An engaged representative can advocate for your loved one during a vulnerable period, ensuring timely treatments.[159]

The diseases that cause dementia are often long-term, chronic diseases. Your loved one might be in the early stages for years. If she suffers an unexpected illness or injury during this time, doing everything possible might lead to recovery. The advance directive or living will, in conjunction with a durable power of attorney for health care, provides written preferences along with an advocate to ensure your loved one is treated effectively.

Discuss Possible Future Living Arrangements

If appropriate, discuss his preferences: to stay at home, to move in with you, or to consider a care facility. My father-in-law was adamant. He never wanted to live with his children. Others prefer to live with family. However, while we acknowledge his desires, circumstances might dictate other solutions.

Do not make promises you might not be able to keep. According to James Whitworth, "Never make a promise you cannot keep. 'I'll keep you at home as long as I safely can' is the most you should promise."[160] No one knows the future. While you may desire to keep him at home, what will be best for you and your loved one might point toward facilities suited to meet your loved one's needs.

While a person with Alzheimer's-type dementia might not remember the details, he can emotionally remember and may accuse the caregiver of trying to get him put away, or steal his money. Since many with LBD often remember recent events, he might remember your promise, but no longer have the capacity to understand the reason for the decision.

Discuss the options as a team, focusing on the disease as the enemy, and consider the types of facilities he might prefer. If he is willing, tour some nearby facilities to get an idea of what is available in your area.

Discuss Other Hard Decisions

This is a good time to discuss upcoming changes that will eventually have to be made, such as retiring if still working, or giving up driving. Her acknowledgement that these changes will have to be made often makes it easier for her to accept the change when the time comes.[161]

This is also the time to ask our loved where she wants to be buried, discuss funeral arrangements, and have her prepay the expenses, if possible. Thankfully, I was able to go through these decisions with my mother when she could express her wishes. She wrote out a list of hymns she wanted sung at her funeral. While we were not expecting her to die soon, it was comforting to know these decisions had been made ahead of time.

These decisions help the family cope with the funeral arrangements, even though it's difficult to do. We can answer any complaints by saying, "This was what Mom requested." Since she had prepaid and planned the services, this relieved us of some of the burdens of decision-making after her death.

Help Your Loved One Maximize Her Health

The brain is impacted by the body's overall health. Good diet and exercise, coupled with enough sleep and consistent daily routines, help the brain as well as the body. Exercise gets the blood flowing and opens up the blood vessels. It also stimulates the brain. Eating nutritious, balanced meals; keeping socially and physically active; and continuing to learn, engaging the brain, slows cognitive decline.[162]

Exercise Is King

Recent studies demonstrate that people with dementia who participated in aerobic classes saw improvement in cognitive function and overall mental health.[163] No study has proven aerobic exercise can reverse dementia, but it does help maximize capabilities. Effective exercise is physically demanding, mentally stimulating, includes interaction with others, and is also enjoyable. Find activities your loved one is willing to do regularly, such as dancing or playing a favorite game or sport.[164]

An activity as simple as walking gets the blood flowing to the brain as well as the body. Even rocking in a rocking chair can be beneficial by improving mood and requiring less pain medication.[165] My mother walked up until the last few weeks of her life.

Exercise helps maintain muscle strength and balance. A well-balanced exercise program will help your loved one preserve strength to function throughout the day. Falls are a great threat and can lead to broken bones or hips. If available, a physical therapist can help maximize balance and provide exercise routines to improve posture and walking patterns. Physical therapy that strengthens muscles and improves balance helps prevent falls and slows down decline, making it possible for your loved one to continue functioning.[166]

Diet

We need to ensure our loved one's diet includes lots of fruits and vegetables, along with reducing trans fats (often found in processed foods), and sugars. A heart-healthy diet is also a brain-healthy diet.

As we learned in Chapter 3, while the brain is only two percent of the body, it requires twenty percent of the available energy. As we age, our cells have a more difficult time taking in sugar. Some people find that coconut oil helps give the brain that added boost.[167] This nutritional supplement works better for some, but not for everyone.

Treat Everything

Ensure your loved one is still taking care of his other health needs. If he suffers from ailments, such as arthritis, that produce chronic pain, make sure he remembers to take the medications for these issues, as well. As his ability to communicate is compromised, he will eventually reach the point where he will have trouble identifying where the pain is. Eventually you will need to give the pain medications without his requesting them.

Help Your Loved One Fulfill Life Wishes

People in the early stages of dementia can remain active and productive for years. Two recent examples are Dr. Richard Taylor and Glen Campbell. Dr. Taylor, a psychology professor, wrote *Alzheimer's from the Inside Out* and gave lectures for years while living with dementia. After Glen Campbell was diagnosed with Alzheimer's disease, he finished *Ghost on the Canvas*, and with his family's help, completed a 151-event tour performing his music in North America and Europe. A documentary, *Glen Campbell: I'll Be Me*, was made of the family's experiences touring in 2011-2012.

Someone with early stage dementia can still function well in many other areas, even if he has deficits that interfere with daily living. He might not be able to drive himself to a school, but he can volunteer to help young students learn to read.[168] There is much living to accomplish, even with dementia.

Mom always wanted to go places—she had an adventurous spirit. If someone around her talked about going on a trip, she wanted to go, too. We took her everywhere whenever possible. While my parents had already completed their globe-trotting adventures, she had one trip left to take—attending a wedding in Colorado. At times it took longer, but those family trips are now treasured memories with few regrets.

No one knows how quickly our loved one will progress. To delay further might render the activity out of reach sooner than you would hope. Take advantage of this opportunity to help make your loved one's wish list a reality.

Staying active utilizes abilities and stimulates the brain to maintain functionality, often slowing degeneration. These diseases work slowly and many can stay in the mild stages for a long time. There is a lot of living to be done during this period.

Memory Aids

In the beginning, lists, notes and calendars work well. These work as long as she is capable of understanding the notes and can follow instructions. Mom liked to check off each day on her calendar. When I visited, we would go over her notes and add future events. While my friend Carol worked full-time, she and her mother communicated through notebooks. Carol still has these keepsakes of her time with her mother.

You adjust to the changes; you simplify. You live life to the fullest possible with your loved one during the early years. Just as farmers gather in the harvest before the winter, we gather in the last adventures with our loved ones. We can help her tie up loose ends and complete projects.

This only works in the earliest stages. If she insists something is going to happen that is not on the agenda or that happened earlier, you can try to help her understand the truth. However once this regularly leads to arguing, it's time to affirm her emotions, and find points of agreement without lying. We need to refrain from correcting her statements, but let them pass.

When Denial Becomes a Symptom

We need to be ready to identify when dementia has impacted the areas of the brain that lets your loved one know he's not thinking properly. His denial might have developed into more than a psychological coping mechanism. If he does not perceive he has problems, he might not just be avoiding the bad news—he truly believes he's okay. If the areas of his brain used to update his internal self-image are damaged, he might not know he has a problem.

This denial, called *anosognosia,* may worsen as the disease progresses. In the beginning, he might perceive he is forgetting or not thinking properly. As deficits increase, he will become increasingly unaware that his reality does not match the world around him. See the section on Chapter 3: Dementia's Assault on the Brain for more on this issue.

Reasoning will not work. As intelligent as he appears to be in other areas, our loved one cannot adjust his thinking to reality despite the facts. We have to listen to him to perceive his reality. We must rotate to his world and meet him where he exists in his mind.[169] It sometimes feels like stepping through the looking glass into wonderland.

Trying to bring him back to reality usually leads to arguments and reinforces his point of view. Sometimes, we fear for his safety as well as for others. However, in his mind nothing's wrong, so there's no need to make changes.

Anosognosia also occurs with other neurological diseases, such as schizophrenia and bipolar disorder. Dr. Xavier Amador, a clinical psychologist who has dealt extensively with the problem of denial, developed the LEAP® method to help patients accept treatment and solutions.

LEAP stands for Listen, Empathize, Agree, and Partner®.[170] We need to listen to him, even if we know his reality does not exist.

We can find some way to empathize. If he truly believes his wife is cheating on him, we can respond with something like, "I can understand how that makes you feel upset." We need to find common ground. Sometimes, we can distract, redirect, or bring up a task that needs to be done. We seek to find a way to help him move on with his day.

Sometimes, we can meet the underlying emotional needs causing these reactions. He may fear that his wife will leave because of the dementia, and expresses it through his accusations. We can respond in ways that telegraph our love, and help him transition to the next event of the day or his favorite music. In this way, we validate his worth and value. These issues will be covered in greater detail in Chapter 6: The Middle-Moderate Stages.

Jade Angelica, in her book, *Where Two Worlds Touch*, relates an experience with her mother who had dementia that demonstrates reflective listening and finding common ground to arrive at a solution. The doctor had recommended her mother begin taking vitamin B-12 supplements. She tried to buy them for her mother in a local health food store. When her mother publicly protested the purchase, Jade put the vitamins back and they left the store. Instead of confronting her mother about the refusal to get the vitamins, she calmly asked what the problem was. She was surprised to learn that her mother had an issue with the store, not the vitamins. Once she learned her mother preferred to get them from her favorite drug store, the problem was solved. Gentle questioning revealed the real source of the problem along with a viable resolution.[171]

We need to remove ourselves from our own biases, emotional baggage, and fears. When her outbursts bring up past conflicts, it's easy to erect walls and dig in our heels. If we honestly seek to understand and find a workable solution, we can defuse the situation:

- refuse to react negatively
- remove the trigger and defuse the situation
- seek to identify the cause(s) from her point of view
- work with her to find a solution.

This is easier said than done. We are not a third-party nurse or social worker. We have a history with her, whether positive or negative. Old habits can rear their heads. Instantly, we can feel the urge to bite back, insist, and add to the crisis.

This story also demonstrates that while your loved one is having problems in some areas, she can still reason, think, and arrive at conclusions. Even though she might not be thinking clearly in all aspects, we can still respect her by meeting her in her world, by not talking about her in front of her, and by having the courtesy to work with her as much as possible.

This is where, in Christ, we can seek to find new ways to deal with our changing loved one. We can rely on the Holy Spirit to transform our minds to respond in love, not anger (remember Romans 12:1-2). We can still learn new ways, expanding our minds.

A soft answer turns away wrath, but a harsh word stirs up anger.
Proverbs 15:1

Speak Truth in Love

Rather, speaking the truth in love ...
Ephesians 4:15

Ephesians 4:25 tells us to "put away falsehood," and to tell the truth. However, Christ also commands us to speak the truth in love. How we say it is as important as what we say. Love is patient, kind, humble, and considerate. It is not rude, arrogant, pushy, insistent on its own way, or thoughtless (1 Corinthians 13:4-5). Yes, we speak truth, but we do it gently, with reasoned care and consideration.

How we speak the truth in love to her will change as she progresses. In the early-mild stages, there is value in gently helping orient her to reality. However, you will need to look for her viewpoint as anosognosia advances. It is time to orient yourself to her world and validate her emotions when she becomes defensive and upset, and does not appreciate your corrections.

Truth in facts is important, but lovingly speaking the truth is greater. We don't have to correct every statement, we don't have to agree with the facts, but we can find some common ground to carry the conversation forward.

One of the goals of habilitation therapy is to enable her to maintain a positive outlook throughout her day.[172] We look beyond the literal words she speaks to the underlying emotion she conveys. Instead of correcting, we focus on validating her emotions, reassuring her of our love, and helping her feel secure.

For example, we can agree that it is upsetting when a valued object is stolen and offer to help find it. "I understand how distressing it is to lose your pocketbook. Can I help you find it?" we could say, and begin searching everywhere for it (remembering she might have left it in an unusual place).

We all need to give and receive love, feel useful, and express our emotions. When our loved one is disoriented to time and less able to rely on recent memories for context, her creative mind will call up events from her past where she felt safe, secure, and included.

For example, what do we tell her if she refuses to eat supper until her husband comes home from work even though he has been dead for years? How do we help our loved one stay calm and happy even if she no longer understands or remembers the loss of her husband? What is the harm of creating little lies to help her get through her moments of confusion?

She expresses her desire to feel safe and a vital part of the family by recalling a distant memory when she prepared the meals for her lifemate. But, the white lie is a quick fix and not a solution. Telling lies does not help meet her unmet emotional needs. While she might not be able to explain it, she could intuit the deception and feel as if you do not take her seriously.[173]

We can try to help her work through the emotions by talking about the loved one. "I remember how you used to love going to the woods for the day and fishing in the creek. We had so much fun." If we can draw out her memories of fonder times and reflect on her lost spouse, we can then help her transition to the next part of her day—setting the table, serving the rolls, and sitting down to the meal ready to eat. Ask her to reminisce about the love of her life. Try to move her past knowing it's suppertime and he's due home from work any moment.

We cannot assume that she's not going to remember the lies—this might be the rare instance when she does remember. I was continually amazed at the facts and statements my mom remembered. If you lie, she might just remember you told her that her husband would be arriving an hour later and wanted her to go ahead and eat. What do you say when he still doesn't arrive? Tam Cummings relayed consequences she observed in her work as a geriatrician. If the loved one remembers your lie and insists on going to find her husband, this can lead to a confrontation.[174] While she might not remember, she's not stupid.

One lie often leads to another. You tell her he called to say he would be late so go ahead and eat. She asks when he called as she never heard the phone ring. You find yourself weaving a series of falsehoods to make your story plausible. Eventually, you might have to inform her that her husband died years ago. This can produce torrents of sorrow as she relives the grief all over again. The better option is to respond to her expressed feelings and not the exact words.[175]

Not orienting her to the reality that she has been a widow for a long time is not deception. We understand she can no longer join us in that reality, but we can meet her in her needs—to affirm her feelings of loss or sadness. She cannot put meaning to her feelings. So, she reaches out for comfort in memories still strong and vivid— the homecoming of her husband to a meal she prepared. We reach past the cold logic of her words to the underlying expression of the need to be loved, and to feel safe and secure.

Our loved ones with Lewy body dementia or frontotemporal-type dementia might not have damage to the section of the hippocampus that produces time disorientation. Not every person with dementia becomes confused about the current decade. However, we need to strive to speak truth in love in all situations. Love covers a multitude of sins and we need to be slow to take offense (James 1:19 and 1 Peter 4:8).

Adjust Situations to Maximize Capabilities

Does our loved one do better with notes than verbal instructions? Can she still handle multistep instructions? Should you take her shopping when the stores are less crowded? Try to arrange schedules so you do not rush her or yourself. Use common sense and your imagination to pick up on your loved one's difficulties, and devise ways to keep her engaged. If noisy spaces now bother her, a change of venue to a smaller, less traveled place might work.

Try to discern if her reluctance to do an activity stems from having forgotten some of the steps. If you help her get started, it might make it possible for her to continue. For example, helping her find everything she needs to mend an apron could be all she needs to sew that day. We might help her participate in conversations if we slow down and take the time to include her in discussions.

Many of your loved one's abilities will remain, such as playing hymns from memory. We need to discover and focus on what she can still do. If she can participate in an activity, even if on a reduced level, she is still maintaining her current level.

From day to day, even hour to hour, our loved one might swing from barely impaired to unable to find her way to the kitchen. Some days the brain struggles to connect the neurons and get the messages across. Stay alert to times of the day when your loved one is usually at her best.

Sometimes, your loved one's personality can shift from a sweet, patient demeanor to curt, insulting insensitivity. Remember, it's the disease producing these changes. Rely on God's grace as you remember how your loved one had been before the disease. With some, the changes might allow personal healing to occur as old controversies are forgotten and your loved one is now willing to accept your help.

Dealing with Apathy

Apathy is common across the diseases which cause dementia. It can be seen in the beginning stages and increases as the disease progresses. It can include a reluctance to begin an activity, the lack of ability to complete tasks, an increased reluctance to talk and interact with others, a lack of understanding of other's feelings, or decreased emotional responsiveness to others.[176]

Described as goal-directed behavior, researchers have identified three component functions: initiation, planning, and motivation. Each function, traced to damage in different parts of the brain, points to different solutions.[177] Helping our loved one overcome apathy involves identifying the underlying components and crafting individualized solutions.

Problems arise when areas in the brain cannot create a signal strong enough to initiate an action. Helping our loved one begin the task often works in the earlier stages. Once we help her get the ball rolling, she can go on to complete the task. When we stimulate as many senses as possible, we can sometimes get the activity rolling. For example, lay out the needed items so she can see them, coach her on the next step, and do the action at the same time.[178]

However, apathy due to planning issues points to problems with thinking and reasoning, remembering the order of the steps, retaining enough information in working memory, or the ability of the brain to select the proper network (such as shifting from the default mode network to the central executive, as explained in Chapter 3). If your loved one has a problem with any of these functions, she will need more help doing the task, to be given one-step instructions (hard to do), or simplified end goals.[179] For example, if she can no longer follow a recipe to bake a cake, she can assist with whipping or mixing as you do it with her.

When motivation is the problem, our loved one's ability to perceive either negative consequences or rewards is impaired. The brain's circuits that motivated her to avoid embarrassment or negative consequences have been impacted. She is no longer internally motivated to placate, appease, or soothe others.[180]

Utilize your knowledge of your loved one's likes, history, and current skills to discover what sufficiently motivates her to overcome her apathy. Studies show that improving the lighting in an area or focusing it on the activity may increase the positive stimulation, increasing motivation. Use of positive encouragement with praise and favorite foods can also encourage your loved one with FTD.[181]

The best care fits the uniqueness of our loved one. One-size-fits-all therapies, which may include music, exercise, pet therapy or specialized care units, have been less successful.[182] We can draw from our knowledge of her likes, dislikes, and what motivates her to act, along with understanding of the disease(s) she has. We can tailor the motivations based on her current likes and dislikes (which can be subject to change as well).[183]

***

In Chapter 1, I told the story of when my mother struggled to organize her sitting room. A month after Mom moved in, I was pleased to see she had organized her bedroom so well. I anticipated she would also create order out of the chaos of her sitting room. We piled the last of her boxes along the long wall of her sitting room so we could accommodate her car in the garage. However, day after day, I saw little progress and grew concerned as the clutter mushroomed, I feared the stacks of unpacked boxes were making it harder for her to set up the room.

I realized she needed more help. I prioritized the boxes and moved the ones full of photo albums, photos, and picture frames into another room. "Let's do it one box at a time," I said, hoping she would be able to handle the more focused task. Mom smiled back and I thought everything was okay.

Then, I noticed she was cutting up envelopes and letters in an attempt to keep names and addresses of family and friends. Boxes and bags of greeting cards were piled precariously around her sitting chair. The box selected for unpacking sat unopened nearby.

She needed help, but I couldn't take over. Setting up filing systems that suited me might not work for her. I didn't have the time to do it for her, and that would not have been good for her either.

I helped as much as I could and tried to work with her attempts to organize. Capitalizing on her efforts, I helped her complete a task and move on to the next step. Eventually, over time, we managed to clear out the space around her computer desk and her chair, but some of her boxes remained unpacked until after her death.

What mattered? Having a neat sitting room with meticulously organized addresses, cards, books, and photos? Time with Mom, with family; time for sitting on the deck eating brats and watching squirrels race from tree to tree had to take priority. As long as she could function, the room was as uncluttered as possible, and she was happy with her sitting room—that was the goal.

<hr/>

We can try to initiate activity, enabling each step if necessary, but we must accept she will be less active. It is a delicate balance between urging her to move and engage versus accepting a decreased level of activity. Neurodegenerative diseases produce lethargy and inertia. If her get-up-and-go decreases, work with her new level. Success is optimizing remaining potential. Remember, it is not rehabilitation to regain former levels of competencies or activity.

Sometimes, we have to be honest with ourselves. Are we willing to let Mom organize her own space, even if it looks messy? Can we accept she now can only play simpler card games and has to give up bridge? We need to adjust to her changing choice of clothes, entertainment, and activities. What matters most is enabling her to stay involved and engaged. We need to be willing to walk with her when she can no longer run. As long as she is still walking, at whatever pace, that is success.

Your Loved One Might Develop Problems with Socialization

Our loved one might misread social situations and respond inappropriately. We might have to be more upfront about telling her when it is time to end a conversation and move on, or redirect her. She might be missing the cues she would have noticed before.

Give her praise and encouragement to be polite and thoughtful. Studies with Alzheimer's patients discovered consistently rewarding good behavior helped them maintain social skills.[184]

My sister Joan encountered this when my mother stayed with them for a month. Joan told me, "She became less and less aware of being considerate of others. The girls would be doing home schooling. If they came into the kitchen where she would be sitting, she told the same stories over and over, and talked for a long time. They had to get back to school. Eventually, they tried to avoid the kitchen. Mom was really unaware that they had work to do; unaware that she had told the story before. Bless her heart, she wanted to interact, but those social cues that said 'I need to get back to my work' just weren't there at all."

What to Do When Your Loved One Does Not Recognize You

Particularly with Alzheimer's-type dementia, she might eventually forget who we are to her. While, emotionally, she knows she can trust us and will often greet us warmly, intellectually, she might not remember our names, or that we are her child.

If your loved one becomes confused and agitated, believing you are an imposter in her house or driving the car, step away for a while and return. This worked for Lela Shanks, a civil rights activist whose husband had Alzheimer's. One day, her husband came into the kitchen and did not recognize her. Thinking she was an imposter trying to break up his marriage, he began yelling at her and told her to leave. Lela went through the back door and sat outside for a while, praying and calling out to God. About thirty minutes later she tapped on the door. He let her in, greeted her warmly, asking where she had been.[185]

This trick also worked for my friend Carol on a long road trip with her mother. She could not convince her that she was not an imposter stealing her daughter's car. So, Carol pulled into a rest area and went into the bathroom. When she returned, she found her mother talking with her brother who had parked alongside them.

Her mom said, "There you are. I don't know who was driving the car, but she was terrible!"

Carol laughed, relieved that her mother now recognized her, and they successfully completed the trip.

Value of Visiting Even if She Does Not Remember Your Name

The fact she feels and these feelings linger long after she has forgotten the events that caused them allows her to give and receive love.[186] The happiness we extend to her with our visits persists past her memory of them. This remains true even when she does not recognize us.

Is there value in visiting her even if she no longer remembers we are family? Yes. Jan Zimmerman, a director of nursing in Watertown, Wisconsin, called it "heart memory. I might not know who you are but, I know you are a good person in my life. You're somebody I want around. I may not be able to say you're my daughter, but I'm happy to see you. It's so nice of this stranger to visit me and you're a safe stranger."[187]

She remains a wife, mother, or daughter, even if how she fulfills these roles has changed. We greet our mother with dementia as our mother. We enable her to connect lovingly with us to the extent of her abilities. Through photos, mementos, or favorite walking trails, we help her remember for as long as possible. As her deficits mount and her abilities to fulfill her social roles morph and change, we walk alongside her. The love we extend to her is never in vain, even if through the ravages of frontotemporal dementia (FTD), she no longer smiles back or hugs us warmly.

Early-Mild Alzheimer's-Type Dementia

Since vascular cognitive impairment often follows a pathway similar to Alzheimer's disease, the two will be considered in this section (see chapter 3 for greater information concerning impeded blood flow in the brain).

Perseveration – Repetition

Perseveration is repetition of an action, story, or question. Patience rules the day. In the beginning stages, perseveration usually occurs because of an inability to retain the answer or remember they already told the story. My mother would repeatedly ask the same question.

Since this is a neutral behavior, not likely to put our loved one in any danger, we can answer a second or even third time; listen to the same story or suggestion over and over. If your loved one continues to be concerned that an event has not occurred or a task has not been completed, in the early stages you may be able to help her remember by asking her to write it down or repeat it to you several times. If this helps them relax, knowing the deed was done, it's worth a try. Mom and I used a white board and calendar to help her remember the week's events. This worked for a while.

In the early stages, while our loved one is still aware and able to adjust, we can help her develop ways to cope with the erosion of recent memory. Walking beside her, we enable her to remain as independent as possible. However, we need to be on the lookout for signs it's time to shoulder more burdens. Hopefully, she willingly transfers responsibilities to us, passing on the torch.

Overcoming Apathy in the Beginning

If our loved one is less active or participating less in conversations, we should try to discern the root cause: can she complete the task once we help her start it, can we structure the social setting or conversation in a way that helps her participate in the discussion, do we have to simplify the steps or do part of it for her? Success can be measured by seeing an action done. She can also achieve it if we lower the bar. Perhaps, she no longer needs to perform at her former level. If we can find a way to keep her involved, that is still a win.

***

We set up Mom's computer in her sitting room. My husband Ralph put her email icon on her desktop and made sure the computer would automatically activate her email account when it was selected. Thinking she was good to go and could continue to email, we told her everything was ready.

A short time later, Mom asked me for help emailing. After frustrating ourselves and her with attempts to "teach" her how to email, we finally realized she was not able to email on her own. The short-term solution involved getting the computer ready so she could sit down and compose a message to her grandkids or friends. Once she wrote her message, I sent it for her. I had to accept this was the only way she could continue to email.

She could no longer email anytime she wanted to. But, she could still converse with friends and family with my assistance and that was the main goal. That first Christmas Mom lived with us, she wrote a beautiful Christmas letter, informing friends and relatives of the latest twists in her life. Even though she needed help with the formatting and printing, it was still her letter.

***

Part of dealing with apathy is understanding and accepting that she might not need to do everything she used to do at the same level. Even though we want to help her do all she can at the time, we need to accept her current limitations.[188] Her value and worth does not rest in her accomplishments.

Our Loved One May Experience Sudden Mood Swings

In her book, *Your Names Is Hughes Hannibal Shanks*, Lela Shanks described how he would swing from laughter to spontaneous weeping, unable to explain the reasons for the outbursts.[189]

If our loved one is at a loss to explain sudden intense feelings of sorrow or joy, we can affirm his emotions. Remember, we should "rejoice with those who rejoice, weep with those who weep" (Romans 12:15). Rely on the Holy Spirit to help us come alongside. We can walk with him through the sudden emotional swings. He doesn't have to explain why he is sad.

Our Loved One Might Become Lost

Our loved one may experience disorientation in the early stages with Alzheimer's-type dementia, and get lost. She might lose her inner maps telling her where she is and where she needs to go. If she is confused, she might not remember her name or address. Since this can happen without warning, an identification bracelet with name, address, and contact telephone number with some mention of dementia, can help her get back home.

Organizations such as the Alzheimer's Association have a Safe Return® program. Check with your local law enforcement office for policies for those with dementia. Some offices will add the information to their database, or even run a dedicated program for helping people who wander or get lost.

If she experiences increasing incidents of getting lost, you may need to make changes: she may require constant supervision, may need to stop driving, or probably should not live on her own. Once your loved one reaches this point, you must remain vigilant to keep her in sight when out and about. She can disappear quickly, even if you leave her alone for just a moment.

Early-Mild Frontotemporal Dementia (FTD)

FTD starts with the frontal or temporal lobes, leading to behavioral, emotional, or speech problems. The most common type—behavioral variant (BvFTD)—may develop in people still in the prime of life, in their forties or fifties. Many of them have children in the home, as well as living parents. Since many of the fundamentals for dealing with behaviors are similar amongst the various diseases, this will be covered in the next chapter, Chapter 6: The Middle-Moderate Stages.

Pursue the Correct Diagnosis

Since FTD can strike those under sixty-five and often begins with behavioral and emotional problems, misdiagnosis is common. Some people are diagnosed with depression, bipolar disorder or another psychosis, Alzheimer's disease, or dismissed as simply under too much stress or going through menopause. The slow, insidious nature of FTD may be misidentified as a temporary deepening of your loved one's standard quirks and personality traits.[190] In the past, your loved one may have been prone to hold grudges or imagined slights. Therefore, doctors may overlook current actions, and don't recognize that the incidences of the behavior are increasing. This can lead to the dementia not being diagnosed until later in the earlier stages. Persist until you find a doctor who hears, listens, and respects what you are saying.

Without the proper diagnosis making it possible to choose disability or medical retirement, some experience devastating financial losses along with losing their careers. For example, a physician with undiagnosed FTD may begin missing key details in his diagnoses, and start yelling at patients or approaching them inappropriately. He could be barred from seeking an early retirement or medical disability. Even though he may seem fit and healthy in many ways, he might have progressed past the point where he should be in charge of his own finances or living alone.

Misdiagnosis can also lead to taking ineffective medicines. Many Alzheimer's drugs offer little help with FTD. Len Strickler's wife finally received the proper diagnosis and the doctor corrected her medications. He gladly stopped buying the expensive Alzheimer's drugs. He created a series of excellent caregiving videos that you can find on YouTube.[191]

Before your loved one receives a diagnosis, he might have alienated family and friends, lost his job and livelihood, and greatly harmed his finances.

FTD Apathy

Another devastating aspect of FTD is the type of apathy it produces. Reluctance to participate, and inability to initiate actions or follow through occurs due to difficulties with thinking and reasoning.

However, bvFTD apathy also affects the emotional and motivational centers of the brain. The loved one no longer knows how to respond appropriately or extend empathy to friends and family. Your loved one may develop emotional blunting which includes decreased ability to express emotional warmth, empathy, or concern. Damaged neural circuits in the brain's reward centers decrease the inner pain of embarrassment or displeasing others. Remember, this is not personal or intentional on your loved one's part.

One woman's family were initially confused and upset by her inability to show any love or affection while her cognitive abilities seemed untouched. She no longer reacted in any positive way to her family. Her husband stated, "My head knows this is part of the disease, but my heart—my heart. Why doesn't she love us anymore?"[192] The smile, the glint in the eye, the warmth that many with other dementias can express even in the severe stages, often disappears in the earlier stages with FTD.

It's easy to focus on the outward expressions of personality. We know her ready smile, kind gaze, outstretched hand, and hug. Do we love her because she loves us—and acts like it? Can our love for her survive the loss of these outward expressions?

Paul said, "For while we were still weak, at the right time Christ died for the ungodly. For one will scarcely die for a righteous person—though perhaps for a good person one would dare even to die—but God shows his love for us in that while we were still sinners, Christ died for us" (Romans 5:6-8).

While we were still sinners—God's bitter enemies—Jesus Christ, the Son of God, took our place and our punishment. He paid the ultimate sacrifice that we all might be one with the Father (John 17). Remembering His love, grace and mercy, can we, in turn, extend Christlike love to our loved ones who sometimes behave as our bitter enemies? We can with the power of God.

The behaviors hit hard and fast with FTD. They come earlier than with the other diseases. The loss of care and concern from our loved one makes it doubly hard. The challenge is to believe and understand this is not a choice. He is not choosing to be thoughtless or cruel, but no longer understands the import of his behavior. From early on, he loses the abilities to interact in socially acceptable ways.

Don't be discouraged if you feel you are facing an impossible mountain. Studies show greater anxiety and distress caring for a loved one with bvFTD than with Alzheimer's disease or some of the other types of FTD.[193] The difficult behaviors coupled with mostly intact memories, verbal fluency, and physical capabilities make it hard to cope with, as well as to understand and accept.

FTD Perseveration

FTD can produce compulsive behaviors that the loved one finds hard to stop. Your loved one may binge eat certain types of food, such as sweets; repeat a set of actions; or walk continuously. Having lost his social constraints and impulse control, he acts out what he is thinking at the moment. Even in the midst of an important discussion or event, he will leave to get food to satisfy his hunger. If he likes to keep things neat, he could compulsively stack and straighten everything in sight, without understanding he's trespassing or stealing.

Compulsive behavior is one of FTD's expressions of perseveration. The brain gets stuck in a loop. It's similar to getting a tune stuck in your head. Some people with FTD will walk throughout the day. However, this roaming is purposeful, unlike with Alzheimer's. Finding ways to safely let him walk helps relieve tension and stress.[194] Perseveration can also be caused by restlessness or stress in the environment, such as too much noise or commotion.

Establish a Support Network Early

Studies found that the apathy expressed with FTD, especially the behavior variant, can create difficulties in a marriage. Caregivers experience more stress, depression, and burnout when their loved ones are apathetic.[195] Remember, his actions have changed due to damage in his brain.

Try to step back emotionally and remind yourself of your mission to comfort and care for your loved one. Taking the third-person objective stance of "caregiver" helps. You choose to love him; you decide to act on this choice knowing God in heaven enables you to love.

Develop a network of people who can affirm your efforts to help your loved one. Some areas have support groups dedicated to caregivers coping with FTD. You are not alone. Even if FTD groups are not available, other support groups for dementia would still be helpful.

Seek the Lord and His Holy Spirit for comfort and the ability to persevere. Take all your cares to Him in prayer and look for His answers. If He led you to serve as the caregiver, He will provide the resources. You are not less important than your loved one with FTD. Bring all your frustrations and upsets to God in prayer. Isaiah said, "You keep him in perfect peace whose mind is stayed on you, because he trusts in you" (Isaiah 26:3).

Caregiving at home can be stressful, especially if behavior issues arise early. Respite care might be necessary to get some time away for yourself. If others are willing to help, make specific requests, such as accompanying your husband on walks. When the FTD diagnosis comes after the disease has progressed, he might need to go to a care facility.

Blame the Disease

When he looks so fit and healthy, it's hard to comprehend his brain no longer correctly processes events occurring around him. Arguments, counseling, or lecturing on proper behavior will not change him. He can no longer adjust.

Some caregivers have printed cards explaining the disease that they can hand out when their loved one is causing a problem in public. The FTD Support Center provides various cards on their website that you can use to educate people about the disease. For example, a card might say, "My spouse has a brain disease called frontotemporal dementia. Thank you for your patience."[196] One woman made arrangements with a local store to cover the cost of any items her husband shoplifted.[197]

Even if the family understands these diseases and their loved one's behaviors, friends, co-workers, distant relatives, and neighbors may not comprehend the reality. In Christ, we can forgive and be slow to take offense. If others distance themselves, we must let them go without bitterness or resentment. We will have more than enough to deal with on our own. Ultimately, we will discover new friends and realize who our real friends are.

Many caregivers regret that they scolded their loved one before they understood that the behaviors were caused by a disease.[198] While we cannot do anything about the past, we can determine to do better in the future and seek to find creative ways to channel our loved ones' actions. This will be covered in greater detail in Chapter 6: The Middle-Moderate Stages.

Identify and Work with What Your Loved One Can Do

Work with him to identify activities he can still perform. This might mean accepting doing the task at a lower level. Find the barriers keeping your loved one from participating. Simplifying the activity or providing step-by-step instructions might help him. Since FTD often strikes at an earlier age, your loved one might be healthier with more energy than those with other types of dementia.

If the FTD begins in his left temporal lobe he will have speech problems. When one avenue or method of communication is affected, other pathways might still work. One patient stricken with this type of FTD lost the ability to speak while he could still read and write. His family adjusted to the changes and was able to communicate with him.[199] Try other things, such as pictures, flash cards, or writing in notebooks.

Identify When He Can't Go It Alone

The degree of reasoning impairment and decreased impulse control might render him unfit to manage his own finances, to continue working, or to live independently. His lack of fear, coupled with lack of awareness of these deficits (remember anosognosia), can lead to risky financial behavior such as gambling, susceptibility to scams, binge shopping, or risky investing.[200]

It can be challenging to get him to agree to changes in these areas. Eventually, you might have to limit his access to money or the internet.[201] Giving your loved one a little cash (as much as you can afford to lose), along with some measure of control might help ease the transition.

Each person's situation is unique and no single answer will work for everyone. Rely on God's wisdom and creativity, along with His provisions. Try all avenues available, test every door. "Ask, and it will be given to you; seek and you will find … " (Matthew 7:7-8). Seek for the answers to your loved ones' needs as he transitions from independence to dependence. We need to consider creative or novel solutions.

Early-Mild Lewy Body Dementia (LBD)

Fluctuating Awareness

LBD does not follow a defined route. It begins with short, intermittent lapses of cognition and awareness. Like a roller-coaster ride, you never know if he will be awake and alert, or drowsy and confused. As it progresses, his *good times* will shorten and become less frequent. In the beginning, the good times are the norm. The wide fluctuations of LBD mean that intermittent bouts of confusion and behaviors appear with greater frequency for longer periods as this disease advances.[202]

Capitalize on his times of awareness to discuss important decisions. Caregivers have seen greater acceptance of hard decisions if they discussed them during times when they were alert.[203] Over time, the good times will become shorter and less frequent.

Showtime

Closely related to good times is *showtime*. This term refers to the ability of our loved ones to rise to the occasion for brief periods of time, especially when with extended family or at a doctor's office. Friends or relatives may not believe the severity of the symptoms due to this phenomenon. The effort required to socially participate can be marshaled for short periods of time, only to revert to "normal" levels once the need passes.[204]

Even though it can be frustrating that our loved one can converse well with her son, but barely speak after he leaves, we must recognize that our loved one does not choose to be difficult with us. Some families deal with this by keeping daily logs of the loved ones' actions; others ask a knowledgeable doctor or medical professional to talk with family members.[205]

Medications

Many of the drugs developed for Alzheimer's are also effective with Lewy body dementia. It is important to work with physicians who understand the best medications for the various types of LBD. Since it is closely related to Parkinson's, people can exhibit dementia symptoms only, gradually showing more movement problems, or a combination of both, or mainly Parkinson's with dementia emerging later. Each variation responds differently to medication.

Additionally, people with LBD can suffer poor or even fatal reactions to certain types of drugs. A *Caregiver's Guide to Lewy Body Dementia* has an extensive section on the best medications versus the most dangerous ones for LBD.[206] Some regions utilize a team of physicians in caring for LBD: a general practitioner, family doctor, or internist makes the initial diagnosis; a referral to a neurologist narrows down the diagnosis based upon tests, scans, and observations of behaviors; a geriatric psychiatrist prescribes medications to deal with the varied symptoms.

Treating LBD is a delicate balance between choosing cognitive functionality versus improving movement. When dementia occurs along with muscle spasms, rigidity, or slow movements, the drugs that reduce dementia can increase movement problems. On the other hand, reducing the Parkinsonian symptoms can increase confusion.[207]

Keep a log, especially noting periods after a different prescription is taken or an adjustment is made. The rule is to start low and go slow. Try to add only one new drug over a period of time. Watch for any changes in symptoms during the weeks after your loved one starts a medication. The effects can build up over time, so a new symptom could be caused by a drug started the month before. Additionally, as LBD progresses, the effectiveness of medications also changes.

Hallucinations

Visions, sounds, or aromas can be hallucinated. While they can be treated with medication, work closely with the doctor. The hallucinations often occur earlier in the disease while your loved one can still comprehend that these visions or sounds do not exist. Discuss them with him. Many people with this type of dementia do not find the hallucinations disturbing.[208]

Some medications can help, but make sure they do not produce unwanted side effects. Changing the environment, such as covering mirrors or removing the items that trigger the visions might help. Hallucinations returning could mean the medication is not as effective as it used to be, your loved one might have an infection, or is dehydrated.

Internal Systems Affected by LBD

LBD also impacts the autonomic system that regulates the body's internal systems, such as digestive and vascular systems. This can lead to problems with fluctuating blood pressure or heart rate, constipation, and nausea. Since LBD slows everything down in the brain, this also slows down the intestines. Add fiber to the diet, reduce or eliminate medications that cause constipation, and serve smaller meals more frequently. These help reduce constipation along with the related nausea.[209]

Watch closely to see if your loved one tends to pass out unexpectedly when trying to stand. While this can be more common for the middle stages, stay alert for sudden lapses of consciousness while progressing through the earlier stages. His slower autonomic system needs more time to adjust blood pressure throughout the body when standing up after lying down or sitting. One family discovered that their loved one needed to sit on the side of the bed for a while before standing up to prevent sudden fainting and falling.[210] The biggest issue with fainting is injuries from falls.

Work with a physician knowledgeable about LBD for stabilizing blood pressure and heart rate. Take sensitivities or possible catastrophic reactions to common drugs into account when you choose the proper medications to treat these issues. If your loved one becomes more sensitive to certain medications, you might need to reduce the dosages.

Procedural Memory and Task Sequencing Problems

While he will remember recent events and conversations, and can often recognize family members, he may forget critical steps for activities and the proper sequence of the steps. For example, put water and coffee into the coffee maker, then position the carafe before the brewing cycle begins.

Look for the reasons he feels reluctant to engage in an activity. If you can identify the steps he forgot or their order, you can discover ways to help him complete tasks successfully. Adjust the task to fit his current cognitive level to keep him engaged, even if it's not usually something done by someone his age. For example, if he cannot use tools for woodworking projects, he might be able to sort or stack wooden blocks.

Importance of Exercise, Movement, and Physical Therapy

Since LBD is closely related to Parkinson's, your loved one might develop some movement difficulties. Be on the lookout for rigid, slow movements, balance problems, tremors, or walking difficulties. Regular exercise, including fun activities such as dancing or golf can help maintain functionality. Walking remains beneficial throughout the journey. Many individuals can walk until the end.

Physical, occupational, and speech therapists can utilize abilities to prolong functionality.[211] Keeping your loved one active in one area also benefits other capabilities. Help your loved one improve their balance to prevent falls and the accompanying injuries; speak loudly enough to be heard in a group to maintain social interactions; walk to the dining room, bathroom, and living room to maintain daily activities. Find ways to reduce stress, establish daily routines, remove clutter in the home, and take advantage of your loved one's best moments.

Hard Decisions in the Early-Mild Stages

Many decisions that come to a head at the end of the early stages: stepping down from a demanding job, giving up driving, or not being able to continue to live alone. Once dementia has been identified as the problem, other changes force themselves upon the family.

If at all possible, ask someone else in the family or an authority figure, such as a medical doctor or official, to present this advice or enforce the decision instead of the primary caregiver.[212] If she associates the primary caregiver with the loss of home, car, or job, she might later turn against the caregiver, which may require a change in the primary caregiver. While recent memory is affected early on with Alzheimer's-type dementias, this is not usually the case with Lewy body or frontotemporal dementias. She might remember the one who's responsible.

Handing over Control of the Finances

It is difficult to accept dependence after a full life, including relinquishing control of the pocketbook. It depends on the family's dynamics. The transfer of responsibility from parent to child can be more difficult, however. If no family member is suitable or willing to handle the finances, a court-appointed guardian can be selected (this carries its own set of difficulties).

Try to start the process in small steps. Offer to balance the checkbook, set up automatic bill pay, become the contact person for billing, and handle online access to bank accounts.

Keep an eye out for spending habits and withdrawals. Look for signs of compulsive shopping or hoarding money throughout the house. Eventually, you will have to assume total control of her finances when she can no longer manage them.[213]

During the interim, ensure she has spending money. It will give her a sense of control and can help ease the transition.[214] One husband made an arrangement with his wife's hairdresser to accept the voided checks she was given by his wife and he paid the beautician separately. Even though his wife could no longer write out a check, handing a check to her beautician helped her feel independent.[215]

Retiring or Stepping Down

As head woman's basketball coach for Tennessee University, Pat Summitt had a demanding and influential job. Her doctors recommended that she gradually reduce her role at the university as opposed to complete termination. Working with the university, she stepped aside and accepted the position of coach emeritus. She could still lead and motivate without the stress of direct coaching.[216]

A less demanding job might not be available or advisable, and could adversely impact benefits. Perhaps, your loved one could transition to volunteer activities following complete retirement. It might work better for her. Investigate local volunteer activities. Dr. Whitehouse encourages some of his dementia patients to volunteer at a local intergenerational school.[217]

A medical diagnosis might be required to secure benefits. If your loved one has not reached standard retirement age, he should be able to qualify for disability benefits once diagnosed. The Social Security Administration created the Compassionate Allowance Initiative to fast track disability claims for people with specific types of diseases, including the major diseases causing dementia.[218]

Stopping Driving

Giving up driving is one of the hardest decisions. It represents the ultimate loss of control in a person's life.

However, safe driving requires the ability to coordinate multiple bodily systems as we correctly interpret the world rushing past us. While our loved one's learned responses might be enough in the normal course of driving, she might not be able to react quickly enough when an emergency arises.[219]

Discuss this early after the diagnosis. Ask your loved one who to give the car to when the time comes. Talking about it will help when the time arrives to hand over the keys.

Offer to take her places (you or someone else does the driving), emphasizing that any items she may need will be available. Help her understand she no longer has to worry about getting lost, and someone will always be there to help her out of the car (along with her walker).

Provide transportation to the doctors and her favorite stores even

Dementia Caregiving from a Biblical Perspective

after she can no longer drive. If you can't always do it, find volunteers to fill in. Be prepared for her to bring up the loss of her car. She most likely does not understand (due to the unawareness of anosognosia) why she can no longer drive.

Some states allow a doctor or motor vehicle department to suspend or revoke driver's licenses. Ask someone other than the primary caregiver to discuss why she can no longer drive. Then, take the final step of disposing of the car or taking their keys. If you can sell or give the car away, do it. That removes it from her reach. You may need to take away the keys or disable the vehicle if you still need the car. Lela Shanks replaced her husband's car key with another similar-looking key. When his key could not start the car, she offered to drive and he traded places with her. In time, he automatically went to the passenger seat, allowing her to drive without protest.[220]

Despite the difficulties, we must remember what could happen if she continues to drive. She could cause an accident that could kill or maim her as well as others. Empathize with her feelings of loss of independence and find ways to maintain her dignity, but don't back down. Find alternate solutions for her transportation needs.[221]

<hr />

My sisters and I agreed it might not be a good idea for Mom to drive. She had been at Sienna Crest for a while and had successfully driven to nearby stores. However, we were afraid she might get lost. I tried to accompany her on shopping trips, including doing the driving. As it grew more difficult for her to get her walker into her car by herself, she usually agreed to let us drive.

My sisters also witnessed some poor decision-making while Mom drove. Adding up all the facts, we told her that her oldest granddaughter needed a car to go to college. Mom offered to give the car to her. However, she grew reluctant as the day approached.

Joan brought Mom out to her car and she tried to start it. She could not operate the car because she had forgotten how. This helped convince her to sign the car over.

I repeated my promise to take her shopping whenever she needed anything. Often, I compiled a list and brought her the items since it was easier than her having to walk through the stores. While it sometimes felt she always had another list the day after I shopped for her, this was far better than taking the risk of allowing her to drive on her own.

Even though Mom had been happy to give her car to her granddaughter, she still talked about missing it. We acknowledged her feelings and agreed it was hard to let the car go. I set aside my feelings of guilt, and commiserated with her over the loss of her car. As time went on, she mentioned the car less and less.

Sidebar: Signs It's Time to Stop Driving

Driving is a privilege, not a right. It's earned by demonstrating the knowledge, skill level, and experience necessary to safely operate a vehicle. In some states, you could be held legally responsible for his accidents if you were aware he lacked the capacity to drive safely and you took no action to block his driving.[222]

Warning Signs:

Trouble with short-term memory, losing the ability to remember road signs or directions

Problems with reading comprehension, leading to difficulty understanding road signs

Cannot react quickly enough to unexpected situations due to slow thinking processes

Exhibits poor judgment, such as pulling in front of other cars or driving the wrong way on one-way roads

Trouble with visual perception, limited field of vision, or trouble focusing near and far (have to be able to read the car's dashboard and still keep track of the road)

Trouble following directions or forgets the proper sequence of steps, e.g. use a turn signal before turning

Slow bodily movements[223]

No Longer Safe to Live Alone

While this occurs earlier in the process with FTD, everyone with dementia will eventually lose the ability to live alone safely. Can she manage a home with yard and garden as she used to? Does our loved one leave the stove on or boil water away? Is she wandering or persistently calling you? Is there spoiled food in the fridge, her clothing dirty or unkempt, or the house unusually messy or in disarray?[224]

Discuss options during the early stages of dementia. Would she like the community of an assisted-living association? Would it work for her to move in with family to enjoy her remaining years with them?

Helping her remain where she chooses for a little while longer might be a good option—for the present. Her last summer at home might be a gift the family can treasure in the future. For the short term, brief frequent visits, home health services, meals delivered to the home, or a monitoring system might work.[225]

Eventually, she will need more care and supervision. How do you know when it's time? When you worry if she has fallen and can't get up; she can no longer manage her own finances or daily routine; she cannot remember where she went or what she just did; it appears she is skipping meals, not taking her medications properly, or forgetting to take them. Each person is unique and the warning signs will differ.

Consider these options: asking someone the family trusts to move in with your loved one; moving her in with you; or moving her to a residential facility. There was a time when multiple generations routinely lived under one roof. Small, close-knit communities, consisting of connected neighborhoods, provided ample resources for helping with caregiving burdens.

Fast forward to today. We are scattered, with most members of the household working jobs away from home. When Mom moved in with us, she was alone for hours while my husband and I worked. We knew few of our neighbors and could not call on them for help. Our children did not live nearby, and our extended family ranged from the East Coast to the Colorado Rockies. Mom spent most of her days alone in her room or wandering the aisles of a nearby Walgreens, often talking with the pharmacy techs.

Think through your lifestyle and your family's needs. Will your loved one be able to make the adjustment if your household includes three rambunctious teens? Is your home rigid or flexible, laid back or more structured? Does the tenor of your home fit your loved one's needs?

After contemplating our home, I realized my mother's outgoing, gregarious nature came alive with social interaction. She loved people and needed opportunities to interact and be a positive influence. She felt dumb and left behind in our house. At Sienna Crest, she found a community where she could love and impact others. My mother blossomed in the right assisted-living facility with the stimulation provided by a community of peers. We still brought her to our house regularly, and included her in family events.

Making these decisions requires prayer and wisdom. Search out the possibilities, keeping in mind that as the disease progresses today's best solution might not be the optimal choice two years from now. Mom's assisted-living facility was small and well-run. As long as she did not require skilled nursing, Sienna Crest could provide care through all the stages of dementia.

Carefully research the various facilities in your area. Don't be swayed by the pretty foyer or furniture. Investigate the staff-to-resident ratios, care complaints, and capabilities. Do they rely on using medications or do they have staff trained for helping people with dementia with a good range of activities? Remember, a good match means the staff will work with you to provide care. Your caregiving does not end; it changes when she moves to a facility.

Go over these options as early as possible. Even if she might forget what you said, she might remember the concept and eventually agree to move to a facility that can meet her needs. While it might seem too soon in the early stages to place her name on a waiting list, it could be a lifesaver if an illness or accident suddenly steepens her decline and she needs to move to a facility. Familiarize yourself with the facilities in your area ahead of time. You will get a better idea of her options and there will be a greater likelihood of an opening for her.[226]

When making the decision, avoid the "should have" thinking. We often believe we should be able to take care of our family; translating into she lives with us in our home. We are not shirking our responsibilities by considering a facility or care community. Taking the third-party, objective viewpoint, we must consider our loved one's needs and safety, as well as our own. Carefully consider the decision to quit a job or career to stay home with Mom or Dad. This often does not lessen stress or avoid depression.[227] It's not always the best solution for everyone. Avoid making decisions out of guilt.

Some caregivers and families have the resources and ability to care for the loved one at home. Utilizing home health care, respite care (such as daycare or short stays in a nearby facility), along with help from family and friends makes it work out. I loved the fact that my mother took care of her Aunt Anna in my parent's home. Years ago, when I visited Mom with my young baby, I could visit Aunt Anna, too. We took her shopping. She adjusted well even though both my parents worked full time. I anticipated we could do the same for my mother, but she was not my great-aunt. She had different needs. My husband and I had a different household with different dynamics. I had to accept the fact that my home was not the best place for my mother.

Whenever these decisions come to a head, remember God will guide you. He provided the perfect assisted-living facility for my mother when she needed a place to stay while we went on our annual scuba diving vacation. It was close by, had a short-term respite care program, and an available room. This became the answer to my prayers concerning Mom living with us. Her time at Sienna Crest for respite care encouraged her to move there a month later.

Sometimes, your loved one will resist needed changes due to the impaired ability to understand it's no longer safe for her to live alone. Begin discussing such changes early, so she has time to adjust to the possibility of moving. Even if she is resistant to moving to a facility or to your home, include her in some of the decision-making: what she brings with her to the facility, and taking her shopping for items she will need in her new home.[228]

Moving to a facility in the earlier stages makes it easier for your loved one to learn the facility's layout and adjust to the staff and routines.[229] By the time Mom slid into the severe stages, she trusted the staff, even if she forgot their names. I had the time and energy to be her daughter, something the staff could not do. Trained professionals helped her with daily problems that I was not equipped to handle. I learned that shortly after Mom moved in. Her back went into spasms and my attempts to make her comfortable made it worse, while it took the aide only a few seconds to ease her pain.

Timing is another factor. Many caregivers can keep their loved one home until the physical burden for caregiving is beyond them. This can happen if you still need to work a full-time job, but she needs more care during the day or she has reached the point where she's awake most nights. No one can keep going, day in, day out, 24/7. Facilities have round-the-clock staffing. As our loved one progresses through her dementia, she might need secure spaces so she can safely wander and not endanger herself. If she becomes bedridden or develops swallowing issues, would you be able to handle it? If you find yourself burned out, stressed, growing angry or frustrated with your loved one, perhaps it is time to consider handing over the day-to-day caregiving to others.

Whatever the solution, the right answer will be the right one for the family at that time. But remember, things can change; they often do.

The Joys and Sorrows of the Early-Mild Stages

You still have your loved one with you for a little longer. Even though a dementia diagnosis is hardly welcomed, finally putting a name to the problem helps. The family can come together and rally around the loved one. During the early-mild stages is the time to visit, go places, and do some of the things that you put off.

I will never forget the trips to the zoo or the mall with my mother, children, and grandchildren. If it was possible, I took Mom everywhere with me. She was there at all the family gatherings for birthdays, anniversaries, and holidays.

I did not have a chance to spend years with the mom I remembered, but I had a chance to spend time with her. She was still my mother and I learned more about her as she changed. My father died within a two-week period—I never got the chance to say goodbye.

Besides the joys of time together, we saw the Lord's answered prayers and the grace He provided in times of need. It strengthened our faith. He is ever faithful.

Eventually, your loved one will slide into the middle-moderate stages with all its hardships and joys. We need not fear because Christ has overcome the world: "In the world you will have tribulation. But take heart; I have overcome the world" (John 16:33). He will not abandon us in the midst of the caregiving call. He is near, very close—we need only remember to call on Him.

The next chapter will look at the middle-moderate stages, where many behaviors and troubling circumstances occur. Remember, no one develops all the symptoms. Each person will have his own subset, which you will learn to know well. Fear not—God will be with you.

---

157 Pat Summitt, with Sally Jenkins, *Sum It Up: 1,098 Victories, a Couple of Irrelevant Losses, and a Life in Perspective* (New York: Crown Archetype, an imprint of Crown Publishing Group, a division of Random House, Inc., 2013), p 375.

158 Joni Eareckson Tada, *When Is It Right to Die? A Comforting and Surprising Look at Death and Dying: Updated Edition* (Grand Rapids, MI: Zondervan Publishing House, a Division of Harper Collins Publishers, 2018), p 161.

159 Ibid., p 162.

160 Whitworth and Whitworth, p 187.

161 Ibid., p 40.

162 Alzheimer's Association International Conference (AAIC), "Going Beyond Risk Reduction: Physical Exercise May Be an Effective Treatment for Alzheimer's Disease and Vascular Dementia." July 23, 2015. https://www.alz.org/aaic/_ downloads/thurs-1130am-exercise.pdf. Accessed 9/15/2017.

163 Ibid.

164 Alzheimer's Association, "Stay Physically Active." www.alz.org/brain-health/
stay_physically_active.asp. Accessed 9/15/2017.

165 University of Rochester, "Rocking chair therapy eases burden of dementia."
www.rochester.edu/pr/releases/med/watson.htm. Accessed 9/15/2017.

166 Heather Cianci, PT, MS GCS, "Chapter 11. A Step Ahead: Exercise and
Mobility," in Gary Radin and Lisa Radin (eds.), *What If It's Not Alzheimer's?:
A Caregiver's Guide to Dementia*, 3rd ed. (Amherst, NY: Prometheus Books,
2014), p 197.

167 I Hu Yang, JE De la Rubia Ortí, P Selvi Sabater, S Sancho Castillo, MJ
Rochina, N Manresa Ramón, and I Montoya-Castilla (2015). [Coconut
oil: non-alternative drug treatment against Alzheimer's disease] [Spanish].
Nutr Hosp Dec 1;32(6):2822-7. www.ncbi.nlm.nih.gov/pubmed/26667739.
Accessed 3/28/2016. Mary T Newport, MD, described how adding coconut
oil to her husband's diet decreased his cognitive disability from Alzheimer's
in her book, *Alzheimer's Disease: What If There Was a Cure? The Story of
Ketones*, 2nd ed. (Laguna Beach, CA: Basic Health Publications, Inc., 2013).
The medium chain triglycerides (MCT) in coconut oil help some patients
with AD.

168 Whitehouse and George, pp 11 and 254.

169 Angelica, p 39.

170 Xavier Amador, Ph.D., *I Am Not Sick, I Don't Need Help! How to Help
Someone with Mental Illness Accept Treatment. 10th Anniversary Edition*,
(New York: Vida Press, 2012), pp 66-69.

171 Angelica, pp 27-28.

172 Deborah Bier, PhD, "Habilitation Therapy for Alzheimer's and Dementia
Care." https://psychcentral.com/lib/habilitation-therapy-for-alzheimers-and-
dementia-care/. Accessed 9/15/2017.

173 Jane Verity, "Truth or Lies—The Great Reality Divide." https://dementiacare
international.com/2007/03/truth-or-lies-the-great-reality-divide/. Accessed
9/15/2017.

174 Cummings, pp 124-125.

175 Ibid., p 125.

176 Devon Schuyler, "Recognition of Apathy as Marker for Dementia Growing."
www.psychiatrictimes.com/articles/recognition-apathy-marker-dementia-
growing. Accessed 9/15/2017.

177 Dr Lauren Massimo, PhD, APRN, Dr Lois K Evans PhD, RN, and Dr Murray
Grossman, MD EdD (2014). "Differentiating subtypes to improve person-
centered care in frontotemporal degeneration." *Journal of Gerontological
Nursing*. 40(10):58-65. www.ncbi.nlm.nih.gov/pmc/articles/PMC4281275/
pdf/nihms 644893.pdf. Accessed 7/12/2016.

178 Ibid.
179 Ibid.
180 Ibid.
181 Ibid.
182 YE Geda, LS Schneider, LN Gitlin, DS Miller, GS Smith, J Bell, J Evans, M Lee, A Porsteinsson, KL Lanctôt, PB Rosenberg, DL Sultzer, PT Francis, H Brodaty, PP Padala, CU Onyike, L Agüera Oritz, S Ancoli-Israel, DL Bliwise, JL Martin, MV Vitiello, K Yaffe, PC Zee, N Herrmann, and CG Lyketsos (2013). "Neuropsychiatric symptoms in Alzheimer's disease: Past progress and anticipation of the future." *Alzheimers & Dementia*. 9(5):602-608. www.ncbi.nlm. nih.gov/pmc/articles/PMC3766403/. "Appendix B: Apathy in the setting of Alzheimer's disease and related disorders: overview and research recommendations," for the Neuropsychiatric Syndromes Professional Interest Area of International Society to Advance Alzheimer's Research and Treatment, by KL, Lanctôt, PB Rosenberg, DL Sultzer, PT Francis, H Brodaty, PR Padala, CU Onyike, L Agüera Oritz, and YE Geda,. Document 2. Accessed 7/12/2016.
183 Rankin in Radin and Radin, p 241.
184 Michael Castleman, Dolores Gallagher-Thompson, PhD, and Matthew Naythons, MD, *There's Still a Person in There: The Complete Guide to Treating and Coping with Alzheimer's* (New York: A Perigee Book, 1999), p 159.
185 Shanks, p 20.
186 Justin S Feinstein, Melissa C Duff, and Daniel Tranel (2010). "Sustained experience of emotion after loss of memory in patients with amnesia." *PNAS* 107(17):7674-7679. www.pnas.org/content/107/17/7674.full. Accessed 9/15/2017. Proceedings of the National Academy of Sciences.
187 Jan Zimmerman, RN, Nursing Administrator, Heritage Homes, Watertown, WI. Interview 5/20/2014.
188 Rankin in Radin and Radin, p 241.
189 Shanks, p 17.
190 Carol F Lippa, MD and Kate J Bowen, "Chapter 7. As the Symptoms Progress: Understanding the Stages of the Disease" in Gary Radin and Lisa Radin (eds.), *What If It's Not Alzheimer's?: A Caregiver's Guide to Dementia*, 3rd ed. (Amherst, NY: Prometheus Books, 2014), p 132.
191 Len Strickler, "Frontotemporal Dementia (FTD) from a Caregiver – Part 1: First Signs." Alzheimer's Support Network. www.alzsupport.org/FTD.html. Accessed 9/15/2017.
192 The Association for Frontotemporal Degeneration, "Emotionally Absent: The Loss of Empathy and Connection in FTD." *Partners in FTD Care*, Fall 2014. www.theaftd.org/wp-contents/uploads/2014/12/PiC-fall-2014.pdf. Accessed 9/15/2017.

[193] E Mioshi, D Foxe, F Leslie, S Savage, S Hsieh, L Miller, JR Hodges, and O Piguet (2013). "The impact of dementia severity on caregiver burden in frontotemporal dementia and Alzheimer disease." *Alzheimer Disease and Associated Disorders*. 27(1):68-73. www.ncbi.nlm.nih.gov/pubmed/22314247. Accessed 6/20/2016.

[194] The Association for Frontotemporal Degeneration, "In FTD, Roaming is Not Wandering." *Partners in FTD Care*, Spring, 2013. www.theaftd.org/wp-contents/uploads/2011/09/spring-2013.pdf. Accessed 4/6/2016.

[195] Massimo, et al..

[196] FTD Caregiver Support Center, "Helpful Ideas—Information Cards." http://ftdsupport.com/side-ideas-buscards.htm. Accessed 9/15/2017.

[197] The Association for Frontotemporal Degeneration, "Hyperoral Behavior in FTD: Changes in Eating and Managing Related Compulsive Behaviors." *Partners in FTD Care* Winter 2015. www.theaftd.org/wp-content/uploads/2015/04/PIC-Winter-2015.pdf. Accessed 9/15/2017.

[198] Len Strickler, "Frontotemporal Dementia (FTD) from a Caregiver – Part 1: First Signs."

[199] The Association for Frontotemporal Degeneration, "Maximizing Communication Success in Primary Progressive Aphasia." *Partners in FTD Care* Winter 2016. www.theaftd.org/wp-content/uploads/2016/01/PinFTDcare_Newsletter_ Winter2016.pdf. Accessed 9/15/2017.

[200] Lauren M Massimo, PhD, AGNP-BC and Geri R Hall, PhD, ARNP, GCNS-BC, FAAN, "Chapter 16. Before Drugs: Nonpharmacologic Approach to Symptom Management," in Gary Radin and Lisa Radin (eds.), *What If It's Not Alzheimer's?: A Caregiver's Guide to Dementia*, 3rd ed. (Amherst, NY: Prometheus Books, 2014), p 248.

[201] Ibid., p 249.

[202] Whitworth and Whitworth, p 49.

[203] Ibid., p 54.

[204] Alzheimer's Australia, "Neuropsychiatric (Behavioural) Changes in Lewy Body Disease." www.fightdementia.org.au/files/helpsheets/HelpsheetLewyBodyDisease03-NeuropsychiatricChanges_english.pdf. Accessed 9/15/2017.

[205] Whitworth and Whitworth, pp 52 and 54.

[206] Chapter 8, Drug Sensitivities and Adverse Reactions in *A Caregiver's Guide to Lewy Body Dementia*, by Helen Buell and James Whitworth, deals with the medication issues regarding LBD, discussing the best and worst drugs. See pages 96-99, 103, and 106.

[207] Ibid., p 65.

[208] Ibid., p 86.

[209] Towne Jennings, pp 78-79; and Whitworth and Whitworth, p 141.

[210] Whitworth and Whitworth, p 154.

211 Alzheimer's Disease Education and Referral Center, "Lewy Body Dementia: Information for Patients, Families, and Professionals." www.nia.nih.gov/alzheimers/publication/lewy-body-dementia/treatment-and-management. Accessed 9/15/2017. A survey of research studies focusing on physical therapy for people with LBD found improvements with physical therapy in the few studies completed so far. Most studies include patients with dementia or movement disorders while excluding those with both symptoms. M Inskip, Y Mavros, PS Sachdev, MA Fiatarone Singh (2016). "Exercise for Individuals with Lewy Body Dementia: A Systematic Review." *PLoS ONE* 11(6):e0156520. doi:10.1371/journal.pone. 0156520. https://www.ncbi.nlm. nih.gov/pmc/articles/PMC4892610/. Accessed 12/5/2016.

212 Whitworth and Whitworth, p 40.

213 Petersen, p 241.

214 Mace and Rabins, p 85.

215 Ibid., p 86.

216 Summit and Jenkins, p 365.

217 Whitehouse and George, p 255.

218 Alzheimer's Association, "Frequently Asked Questions: Social Security Administration (SSA) decision to add early-onset Alzheimer's disease to Compassionate Allowance Initiative." www.alz.org/national/documents/SSDI_ FAQ.Pdf. Accessed 9/15/2017. Frontotemporal dementia, Lewy body dementia, and mixed dementia (including vascular impairment) have also been added to the list. The list is posted on the SSA website (see www.ssa.gov/compassionate allowances/conditions.htm).

219 Mace and Rabins, p 87.

220 Shanks, p 89.

221 Mclay and Young, p 122.

222 Castleman et al., p 225.

223 Leilani Doty, PhD, "Series: Driving and Progressive Dementia, Session 3: Safe Driving and Alzheimer's Disease or a Related Dementia (Memory Disorder)." alzonline.phhp.ufl.edu/en/reading/DrivingADArticleAlzOnlineSess3.pdf. Accessed 9/15/2017.

224 Castleman et al., p 228.

225 Mace & Rabins, p 93.

226 Mace and Rabins, pp 459-460.

227 Ibid., p 362.

228 Ibid., pp 102-103.

229 Ibid., p 104.

6

The Middle-Moderate Stages

During the early-mild stages we helped our loved one function in our world. We provided help and intervention that made it possible for her to thrive in the world. We managed to keep her with us by arranging schedules, driving, gathering the tools and items, filling in the blanks when she lost words, or gently drawing her into conversations.

Each treasured outing, family gathering, completed quilt, lecture, or painting was an achievement we reveled in with her. And, for a while, she could join us in our world. She welcomed the corrections and acknowledged our explanations as she strove to keep up. But then, little by little, she no longer understood the hints or wanted the corrections. She resisted suggestions or changes, digging in her heels just a little deeper.

One day, we understood that her world was not our world, her world was her own. She could no longer come to us, we had to meet her in hers. While it seemed to have happened overnight, she had been revealing this to us, little by little—the time had come to join her in her world.

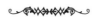

In the beginning, Mom socialized well, was ready when we picked her up for church each Sunday, and regularly consulted her calendar. Since we kept in contact and she came to our house often, I did not feel the need to visit her every day. After all, she enjoyed her friends and the activities at Sienna Crest.

Eventually, however, I realized she no longer connected her calendar with a specific day or time. The page of squares with numbers no longer held any meaning for her. She was not ready Sunday mornings, and telling her of upcoming events made her anxious. On the day I found her wandering the parking lot looking for me to pick her up for the mother-daughter banquet, I realized I had to stop telling her about activities in advance. Whether a doctor's appointment or a family birthday party, I told the staff and showed up early enough to get her ready. She no longer needed me to tell her ahead of time as she had in the past. Now, living more in the moment, she had no trouble going with me without advance notice.

The middle stages require a great deal of caregiver *patience.* Allow time for your loved one to get up or walk across the room, time to get dressed or brush her teeth at the end of the day, to process your question and to answer.

Patience, also known as steadfastness and endurance, refers to continuing on through difficult circumstances. As we know the goal and follow a set course, we continue to love her through all the changes. Even while suffering long, we choose to respond in love. We wait for her to put on her socks, providing aid only if she seems to be struggling and would like our assistance. We answer her question again just as if this was the first time she asked it. We ignore snide comments or insults and continue with the need of the moment.

Through all this, Christ, who endured more than we could ever imagine, will sustain us. We ask Him to share His love for our loved one with us. We patiently persist, knowing love conquers all.

Love bears all things, believes all things,
hopes all things, endures all things.
So now faith, hope, and love abide, these three;
but the greatest of these is love.
1 Corinthians 13:7, 13

Middle-Moderate Stage Considerations

As your loved one transitions into the middle-moderate stages, her current deficits will increase and she will begin to show deficits in new areas. Finding a safe way to help her stay engaged and get through her day with a positive attitude is the short-term goal. As she settles into the middle stages, relying on the comfort of routine helps both of you navigate this period.[230]

During the middle-moderate stages, our loved one might not be able to complete tasks alone as she used to. If she could dress without help when you laid out the clothes, now you might need to show her what items to put on first and assist her in getting them on. She might be able to select her clothes for the day from a small number of choices instead of a full closet. She might be able to set the table if you hand her the plates and utensils. Incontinence could be due to not being able to find the bathroom. Leading her to the bathroom regularly might be all the help she needs. Whatever her particular issues, we need to be alert for her increased need of assistance and guidance, all the while letting her do as much as she can.

Her ways of communicating will morph and diminish. She might begin to use words that don't logically fit what she is trying to say. She might begin to show deficits in new areas such as not being able to schedule events or make decisions. As the cognitive deficits deepen in difficult areas and spread into new ones, our loved one's ability to act as she used to will change. Her emotions might overwhelm her, causing her to lose her self-control, or she might begin to have problems with understanding what she hears or reads.

Our loved ones are trying to connect with us, but the rules

are changing. No longer able to reorient to the world around her, she needs us to learn how to connect in new ways. We can no longer count on our loved one acting in the same, mature, socially acceptable way.[231] We have to start over again because we cannot predict what she is going to do. The rules will continue to transform as her illness advances. The aides at Sienna Crest called this *finding her new normal.*

These changing rules can make us feel off-balance and uncertain how to relate to her. Remembering our decision to love and care for her, we act.

> *An emerging definition of love, then, is an affection,*
> *or a desire for the welfare of another that moves*
> *to a commitment to act for her well-being.*[232]
> Robertson McQuilkin and Paul Copan

Christ called us to love Him with all our hearts and to love others as we love ourselves. We can, and God will enable us to do this since love is a decision of the will. We move beyond feelings. Love acts for the other person in all circumstances.

For example, if our husband with frontotemporal dementia changes how he relates to us, we must understand that he cannot help it—it's the disease. This is when we can rotate to learning how to meet him in his world. Even if his face is a mask and he no longer tells you he loves you, you can love him through Christ, knowing that apart from the dementia, he loves you. This is possible with God's help. We seek to find our "new" loved one, to discover his current likes, dislikes, good times, capabilities, and skills. We seek to learn his new language, perceiving the messages he sends us with his body language, looks, and tone of voice.

We also need to watch our attitude. Sidestepping the temptation to see ourselves as co-victims, just as cheated as our loved ones, we need to focus on Christ. Think back to Philippians 4. Keeping our eyes on Jesus will bring the inner peace that will enable us to sort through the confusion. Instead of focusing on slights, offenses, and what our loved one can no longer do, we need to remind ourselves of our goal to help our loved one live well with dementia. By searching for what our loved one can do today, to the full extent of his capabilities, we become part of the treatment solution. We adjust our attitude and control our emotions, and we try to objectively assess and analyze the situation to solve problems. Improved attitudes enable us to be better caregivers. Our body language and calm intonation will help our loved one remain calm.

In their book McLay and Young said, "A sense of humor acts like a shock absorber for caregivers and loved ones."[233] Laughter releases the tension building up in an awkward social misstep or a dropped cup. Letting go of what used to be—what lay behind us—we press forward to the tasks of the day. If we can see the silver lining, the subtle humor, the soft irony, the little joys and beauty of each day, we can turn an awkward moment into an opportunity to remind him of our love, casting aside pity, anger, and fear.

Our loved one struggles to perceive our needs. Yet, he will still react to our negative or positive emotions. Calm, measured responses from us will help de-escalate the situation. The more we can still our soul in Christ, grounded in Him, the better able we will be to rise to the day's challenges.

Keep in mind that the goal is to help our loved one finish well. Reset goals to match his capabilities—seek the balance between challenging him and what is achievable at his current level. Thinking back to habilitation therapy, we offer failure-free activities that still motivate our loved one to utilize his gifts and talents. We set daily items in order, such as laying out the toothbrush with toothpaste on, ready to go. Plan ahead, to minimize difficulties with dressing, eating, or washing. Anticipate the triggers that bother him, and offer an activity to see if this will be one of his good days. We seek to help him remain calm.

We set in motion established routines to meet the family's needs while maintaining flexibility to capitalize on her good days and adjust for bad days. Seeking the adventure of the day, we find ways to keep our loved ones engaged, while treasuring the time afforded to us.

Middle-Moderate Alzheimer's Type Dementia

Since dementia's progression with vascular cognitive impairment is often similar to Alzheimer's disease, they will be included together (see chapter 3 for greater detail).

Our loved one will continue to have problems with short-term memory, along with increasing disorientation to time and place. She might go from not recognizing you to mistaking you for a lost loved one, such as an aunt or grandparent. She might begin to lose track of the time of day and begin wandering at night or sleeping more during the day. Besides repeating questions and retelling stories, she might also repeat actions or movements. Her ability to find her way to places, such as the kitchen or bathroom, even in her own home, might become compromised. She might have increasing difficulty understanding what someone says to her, correctly expressing her thoughts, or she may begin using inappropriate words, such as swearing.

Middle-Moderate Frontotemporal Dementia (FTD)

The deficits which originally pointed to neurodegeneration in a particular lobe will begin to spread to other areas of the brain. As beginning symptoms become more intense and frequent, new ones also develop. For example, if her deficits began with speech difficulties (pointing to problems with the left temporal lobe), she might begin to have more problems with decision-making and understanding numbers. Your loved one will have increasing problems with impulse control, judgment, and greater apathy.

As our loved one's ability to add emotion to speech and facial expressions, along with being less aware of our emotions, her face becomes more immobile. Some people with FTD might develop an aggressive-looking stare but it will not be motivated by anger.[234] Eventually, her face may not be able to reflect inner emotions. This is called *emotional blunting*.

Remembering how she used to be with us, ignoring the blank facial stares, we smile and encourage her as much as possible. Len Strickler's wife was diagnosed with frontotemporal dementia. In his YouTube videos, he said she responded best when he greeted her warmly and energetically, letting her know he loved her with smiles, hugs, kisses, and positive upbeat energy.[235]

Repetitive behaviors intensify in the middle stages. Your loved one may compulsively walk a particular route, called *roaming*, repeatedly watch the same type of shows, such as game shows, insist on eating ice cream or candy bars throughout the day, or perform activities like ripping paper, doing puzzles, or collecting similar objects. Your loved one's ability to plan and initiate activities may decrease to the point where she can only generate compulsive activities.[236] As long as it can be done safely, find ways to turn the compulsive behaviors into constructive activities. These repetitive behaviors help your loved one relieve the stress of the disease—fold them into her day.

Your loved one might develop swallowing problems if muscle coordination for swallowing and moving food to the stomach is compromised. The biggest issue is aspiration—when liquids or bits of food head toward the lungs and can eventually lead to pneumonia. This can also happen quietly, without initiating coughing or throat clearing.[237] Certain FTD diseases can impede the body's ability to transport food and liquids to the stomach, affecting muscle coordination, the body's ability to interpret taste and sense perception, or increase or decrease saliva production. An increase in saliva, along with swallowing problems, can lead to drooling.[238]

Working with a speech language pathologist or speech therapist can help, as well as requesting nutritional supplements or medications, if necessary.[239] With diseases that begin with significant language impairment, such as primary progressive aphasia, a type of FTD, speech therapy can be helpful.

If your loved one has difficulty with language, she will need more time to understand what you are saying and to respond. We need to slow down in how fast we talk, as well as how quickly we expect a response.[240] The goal is to help her contribute to the conversation.

Select foods that are easier to chew—soft, moist foods that stick together are better than sticky, crumbly, hard, or dry foods. Thicken liquids, chop solid food and cook it until it's soft. Prepare smaller meals throughout the day. Make sure your loved one is not rushed through a meal; ensure she swallows the food before she takes the next bite. Sit up completely. Avoid reclining while eating.

Middle-Moderate Lewy Body Dementia (LBD)

While each person's expression of LBD is different, your loved one's periods of difficulty will become more frequent and last longer. Lucid, alert times still occur, even throughout the later stages. While some symptoms, such as sleep disorders, might now be successfully managed, other issues relating to the body's internal systems or movement problems might intensify or appear. Having trouble seeing, recognizing objects or colors may lead to more spills, stumbles, or falls. LBD slows down the thinking processes, requiring more time for our loved one to respond to questions or move. Problems with movement and coordination may become more of an issue.

Your loved one with LBD may have increasing problems with swallowing. Work closely with your medical team to discover the underlying causes for these problems. Swallowing issues can be caused by neurological problems, muscle weakness, variations in saliva, or a combination of all of these. The solutions might vary, depending upon your loved one's unique expression of LBD. If the timing or strength of the muscles, valves, and sphincters that control the movement of food through the digestive tract are impacted, food or liquids could end up in the lungs, leading to infections.[241]

While memory problems occur, they are most often related to problem-solving and remembering how to do things (forget the order of steps to complete a task). Many people with LBD retain their short-term memory, do not become disoriented to time or place, and continue to recognize family and friends.

Dealing with Behaviors

Eventually, as the cognitive deficits spread, most dementia patients will develop behavioral issues. While these issues usually arise in the middle stages, they can occur earlier with some diseases, particularly the frontotemporal type.

Many people with dementia might act in similar ways, but the underlying reasons can vary greatly. In addition, each person may express dementia behaviors in unique ways. Finding a solution requires identifying the root causes. Your loved one's agitated behaviors could signal the emergence of a basic need, such as having to go to the bathroom, feeling hungry, being too hot or too cold, or in pain. Inability to properly process sights and sounds could render large crowds, noisy environments, or well-lit rooms overstimulating, even torturous for her. She could also be reacting to her recognition of loss of control or of not being able to socialize. Any or all of these reasons could cause periods of distress exhibited by pacing, lack of cooperation, or stubbornness.[242]

Some of the causes for difficult behaviors are:

- illness or untreated pain
- communication problems and misunderstandings
- frustration due to not being able to communicate unmet needs
- fear of the dementia and the resulting losses
- not correctly interpreting sights or sounds
- tiredness or overstimulation
- physical issues
- loss of impulse control

Finding the solution requires investigating the causes. Since there is a long list of difficult behaviors and a longer list of possible solutions, this section will highlight general principles for finding ways to help our loved one stay positive and move through her day.

Is the Behavior Really a Problem?

Our loved one has changed, resulting in altered actions, habits, and preferences. When my mother acted differently, the first thing I had to ask myself was: Does it make a difference? Could I adapt by adjusting my inner perceptions and expectations? My previously extroverted mother now preferred to sit by my side at church, instead of learning everyone's name, networking, and sharing the latest stories. Instead of interacting between services, she sat as the conversations flowed around her. This was her new activity level.

As we meet her in her world, we adjust our expectations to our loved one's new normal. Whether she has become more irritable and easily offended, or more quiet and docile, we continue to interact with love.

Some accommodations I had to make included accepting my mother's changed appearance. As a professional, she kept her hair colored and permed, dressed smartly, and attended to her grooming. Over time, she stopped coloring or perming her hair, didn't mind if she wore the same clothes every day, and just didn't want anyone messing with her fingernails. These changes did not make her sick or put her in danger, so I honored the woman she had become. Her white hair no longer took coloring or perming well; she felt accepted at Sienna Crest, and no longer cared to shop for clothes. She was happy, so I learned to be content with these changes.

Repetitive behaviors can be annoying. I have a bad habit of ticking pages while I read a book. Knowing this bothers my husband, I can stop it when he's around. If our loved one has gone past the point where she can anticipate and extinguish annoying actions, we can ask the same question—is the activity dangerous, or could it have some positive effects? At least she's moving. Can I utilize these actions to help her feel engaged and useful?

If we can perceive the underlying emotion driving the behavior, we should attempt to meet her emotional needs.[243] In some instances, repetitive behaviors can calm our loved one, particularly with FTD-type dementia. Trying to stop the actions could create agitation and distress.[244] We need to remember to blame the disease, not our loved one.

It is okay to acknowledge our inner sadness and grief at these changes. When I greeted my mother who no longer cared if her favorite sweater was stained (it had pockets she could fill with cookies, coffee creamer packets, napkins, and bits of paper), I had to remind myself she was safe, she was content, she was happy. Even as we silently grieve when with them, we allow the moment's interactions to command our attention. Can love cover or overlook it?

Keep a Behavior Log

Document the behavior by recording what, where, how, and when. Use the log to figure out why—identify the triggers, determine our loved ones unmet needs, or devise ways to divert or distract. As the dementia progresses, your loved one will have increasing difficulty communicating needs—such as going to the bathroom, controlling impulses to say or do whatever comes to mind, and interpreting what is going on around her. As we try to see things through her eyes, feel what she feels, and attempt to enter her world to understand the problem, we can begin to craft a solution.

Note the time(s) of day when the behaviors begin. Does it occur in the mornings or late afternoon, or does it go on most of the day? What happened just before the event? Was there noise, did she just finish watching a television show or movie, did someone just walk into the room? Jot down every item you notice, and look for a pattern. Consider your loved one's actions. Are they favoring a leg and walking with a limp, rubbing an arm, or pacing? Note what worked and what didn't work to extinguish the problem.[245]

If your loved one is still verbal and can answer questions, ask her. Try to find out what happened and what she was thinking. In our example in Chapter 5, Jade met resistance when she tried to buy vitamins for her mother. Once they were settled, she gently asked why her mother didn't want the B12 vitamins. Learning the problem was the store, she found a solution that made both of them happy—they purchased the vitamins from her mother's preferred store.

Write down all the facts and circumstances. It can help you notice patterns that you might overlook in the midst of a situation. It will also reveal trends and document the progression of your loved one's disease. Behavior logs also help to document the effectiveness of treatments. This is helpful for your medical team to optimize therapies for your loved one. It also reveals patterns of behavior not caused by us. Don't take the blame; let this rest with the disease—blame the disease.[246] It helps us get emotional distance so we can begin to find the solution.

Alternatively, the log could pinpoint actions or sequencing we do that inadvertently trigger a behavior. If she recoils every time we touch her arm, we can change our approach. If the tone of our voice, whether too high- or low-pitched, creates havoc, we can try to adjust that, as well. If she does not recognize us and perceives our actions as threatening, she will be merely moving to protect herself. Does she say something that triggers us to respond impatiently or harshly, which leads to everyone having an emotional meltdown?

Ask for Wisdom—Let God Inspire You

This can be overwhelming, but with your knowledge of your loved one's history, likes, dislikes and mannerisms, even with the changes, you are uniquely suited to find solutions.

First, pray, asking God to provide the insights. Judy Towne Jennings, whose husband had Lewy body dementia, would sometimes receive answers to perplexing problems as she journaled to God at night.[247] Share your problems with others at work, with your contacts, support groups, or online chat rooms. God will supply the answer.

Second, set aside past ways of doing things and consider novel solutions. Before, we took our loved one for a drive to reach a destination, such as going out to dinner or to the park. However, now she might be happy just going for a ride with no particular destination or purpose necessary. Keep your eyes open for the solution—it sometimes comes from surprising sources. Do not discount an idea that floats to the top of your consciousness. It just might work.

Third, look for God's answer. The promise in 2 Peter 1:3 stands: "His divine power has granted to us all things that pertain to life and godliness, through the knowledge of him who called us to his own glory and excellence." This is the time to take hold of the promise— all things that pertain to life. Look for God to supply the pathway to lovingly care for your loved one in the moment.

Fourth, take courage and lay aside the fear, knowing God will also enable you to provide the care your loved one's needs.

… let us also lay aside every weight, and sin which clings so closely,
and let us run with endurance the race that is set before us …
Hebrews 12:1

Above all, we must remember to extend love to her with kindness, compassion, thoughtfulness, selflessness, humility, seeking what's best for her. She is losing connections with this world, and may realize this in her moments of difficulty.

Look for Infection, Injury, or Poorly Controlled Pain

After you utilize the behavior log, and find ways to help your loved one get up, dressed, have breakfast, and move through her day, she can suddenly change. Once you recover from the shock, fears, and distress, don't forget that illness, injury, or pain can cause sudden behavioral problems. A frequent cause is urinary tract infections. Injuries you were not aware of, infections, or constipation can also trigger sudden declines in behavior.[248]

Keep a Detailed Medication Log

Side effects of medications can lead to behavioral symptoms. The brain, altered by the disease, can make your loved one more susceptible to her medications. Certain medications may no longer be safe or effective. Keep a medication log, noting date, name of drug, amount and dosing instructions, along with physical reactions and new behaviors.[249] Medications may need to be adjusted or dropped. Perhaps your loved one no longer needs the medication or a better option exists.

As your loved one's advocate, you need to stay on top of how your loved one responds to medications even after moving to a facility. You know her complete history, are aware of previous bad reactions to prescriptions.

Medication logs are critical when adding or changing medications. Ask about a drug's side effects and the cumulative effect of the medication. Some drugs slowly build up in the body, so negative reactions might not appear until weeks or even a month after your loved one started taking the medication.[250] If she suddenly behaves differently, think back to any medication changes made over the preceding month.

The Fear, Anxiety Factor

A mature, functioning brain allows us to initiate actions, complete tasks, achieve goals, build dreams, and help our friends and loved ones. To be stripped of these abilities, to see dreams die around us, to grapple with the fact that we will not do more tomorrow than we did today but will cling to what we have as it slips away, touches our inner core. Richard Taylor, in his book *Alzheimer's from the Inside Out* describes it as a primordial fear that permeated his days as he lived with early onset Alzheimer's disease. He likened the fears of dementia to a seething volcano waiting to explode.[251]

Problems with communication, fear or embarrassment at not being able to do what they used to do may cause explosive reactions. Offer patient endurance. Respond with kindness. Extend love. These will help your loved one recover and move on with her day.

Additionally, how we respond to our loved one could also contribute to the conflicts. Our loved one's sensitivity to our emotions can calm or exacerbate the situation.[252] Our loved one still feels, even if she can't identify, name, or express the reasons for her reactions.

As a person, she needs to be loved and validated. We can acknowledge her emotions, even if her facts are wrong. This is not dishonesty when you respond to the reality of her emotions. As we validate her feelings, we extend love to her. Saying yes to her feelings will help her feel loved. Sometimes, a hug or sitting by her side is what she needs.

Crafting the Solutions

Our loved one is the same, yet different. She remains our loved one, yet with new habits, preferences, and needs. Forgetting what lay behind, we reach forward toward the day's needs with new ways of thinking and being. Previously, my mother could verbally connect with people so easily that she did not need hugs or handholding. This changed as her dementia progressed. We learned new ways to be with her, such as sitting close to her and holding her hand.

We reframe how we respond to our loved one. We reassess our roles and responsibilities, taking up new ones as necessary, while never forgetting who she is to us. We repurpose the world around her to hold her safe, calm, and secure.

In order to respect our loved one's dignity, we offer her a choice instead of demanding our way; ask for her to help, even if it's a small thing.[253] Instead of saying "don't" or "no," we shift her focus and then seek to move her toward the next part of her day and away from inappropriate or unsafe activities.[254] Ask her to help you accomplish a task.

For example, while our loved one used to be able to get dressed with little help, this now takes hours. We discover that she gets confused by the choices of a full closet, and her arthritis acts up when she tries to put clothes on. This is the reason she has been resisting our aid; we've been hurting her. So now, we have her eat breakfast and take her pain medication first. Once she feels better, we set out a few outfits on the bed for her to choose from. We gently help only if she indicates she wants the assistance.

The solution could be as simple as rearranging the order of

events, setting up the tools to complete the task, or providing small helps along the way. She might not be able to change how she reacts, but we can adapt. Altering our reactions is the start.

Perhaps her refusal to bathe is due to embarrassment. Your loved one might not resist help with bathing from a third-party professional caregiver.[255]

Next we look for ways to alter her environment. We also can try seeking a therapy or medication solution with the medical team. We find ways to structure her day for success, enabling her to continue to be a part of her community.

Altering Care to Direct Our Loved One's Behavior

How we react to our loved one, our preconceived notions about what our loved one can do, and our attitudes make a difference. Putting our newfound knowledge to work, we can decide to let love cover it; we can respond in loving patience, knowing a soft answer deflects wrath, but responding in kind stirs up anger (Proverbs 15:1). Above all, we can try to not escalate the situation with our own defensiveness, or telling our loved one that she is wrong. Even if we know we did no harm, we can still apologize and promise never to do it again.

Set Routines in Place

As thinking becomes more rigid and inflexible, our loved one may find comfort and security in consistent routines and rituals. We can adapt, adjust, and rotate to create the routines and activities best suited to our loved one's unique lifestyle, preferences, and current cognitive level.[256] Establishing traditions of the day and instilling a set routine to follow as the day progresses allows the loved one to intuit what comes next, relieving stress. The comfort of stability helps maintain positive emotions.[257] Keep things simple and vary the routine as little as possible; develop a daily schedule for medications, meals, naps, exercise periods, bath times, and walks.

Find Ways to Help Your Loved One Rotate to the Next Activity

Look for ways to help move your loved one to the next activity of the day, whether it's time to eat, go to the bathroom, or go for a walk. Invite her to join you or ask for her help. Instead of asking if she wants to eat lunch, escort her to the kitchen and say, "That smells good. Let's have some soup." Stay positive, relaxed and upbeat.

Comfort over Appearance

We remember our loved one's former style of grooming and preferred dress. However, with the changes in our loved one's life, as well as capabilities, the old ways of dressing may no longer fit her current lifestyle or capabilities. Stockings are hard to put on even for healthy adults. Snaps, buckles, zippers, belts, ties, and styled hair might not be practical any longer. The purpose for many of these choices, such as proper appearance for competing in the marketplace and setting a professional tone while working, usually no longer exists.

Now is the time to choose comfort and practicality over appearance and tradition. If our loved one wants to wear the same thing every day, you can wash the outfit frequently or buy multiple sets. If your loved one does not want to change into pajamas at night, let her wear looser fitting sweat suits that are also suitable for sleeping.[258]

Seek Medication Solution Last

Sometimes, medication needs to be considered after all other options have been tried. The mantra is to "go low and go slow"— uses the smallest dose possible. Dosage can always be adjusted as needed.[259]

Set the Stage for Success

Set out the items needed for an activity, being ready for any difficulties. For a time, your loved one will be able to do many things as long as we set out the required items.[260]

Pay attention for signs your loved one is beginning to forget the proper order of steps to do something. Eventually, she will need you to put the items in order of selection or hand them to her one at a time. For example, with teeth brushing, hand her the toothbrush, tell her to get it wet, hand over the toothpaste, and let her put it on the brush.

Communication Basics:

- Make eye contact—ensure you have her attention before speaking
- Speak slowly and clearly with familiar words and short sentences
- Address your loved one directly and don't talk past her to others
- Include her in conversations, assuming she can hear and understand
- Ensure she can hear and see the group
- Don't ask if she remembers or what she did
- Give her clues to aid her understanding of events going on around her
- Give one-step instructions, repeating when necessary
- Try to talk with her in places with fewer distractions
- Respond to her emotions, not necessarily her words, with a calm, gentle voice
- Give your loved one time to respond
- Smile, even if she can no longer smile back
- Give her chances to be in control[261]

Remember, when interacting with your loved one, approach her directly and get her attention—best by establishing eye contact. However, avoid directing from in front or over her. It can be confrontational and make her feel trapped. Instead, once you have her attention, move to her best side. This helps her feel in control, as she can turn away if needed.[262]

Maintaining conversational etiquette, we encourage her to speak and we listen to her; we respond to the emotions she conveys, even if the words lack sense. Matching her expressed mood, whether laughing or sad, we reach out to her in love.[263] Find ways to include her in the conversation by adding hints such as, "Mom, we used to go to the beach and look for clams. Dad always found the most." Talk about the weather or your plans; discuss the holidays and favorite meals or games. By talking about older memories, your loved one might be able to share stories from family events that happened years ago.[264]

Reminding ourselves that love is patient and kind, we seek to make her feel welcomed, included, and wanted. Respect her view of the world, and look for ways to interact and touch her soul.

Stage Appropriate Activities versus Age-Appropriate Activities

Despite her cognitive deficits, our loved one still needs to be active and involved to feel useful and important. However, the activities that she can still do might not match her current chronological age. The trick is to find ways she can participate successfully, which may vary from day to day.[265] Attempt to find activities that are failure free. Include every part of daily life—dressing, bathing, as well as music, arts and crafts, or sports. The positive feelings generated by doing something will help make her day positive.[266]

The right activities depend on our loved one's current stage and her variable cognitive levels. Some days, she will be able to help cook a meal, while other days, setting the table might be the extent of her capabilities. Reacting to her abilities in the moment, we step back and let her do it herself or come alongside with hints, cues, or help.[267]

Try to include activities that involve as many of the senses as possible. It helps keep the brain functioning. Use of art in group sessions helps engage more parts of the brain. Encourage your loved one to discuss what she thinks and feels when she looks at an object or a painting. Some programs enable the loved one to draw a picture as she looks at flowers, a tea pot, or pictures from past events.[268]

Activities that relate to your loved ones past profession might help focus her attention. For example, a former banker or accountant might enjoy sorting money or coins (play money that closely resembles currency works well). A mechanic might enjoy sorting and organizing tools or taking small items apart.

Helping our loved one live well with dementia requires many accommodations on our part. We accept changes in dress, appearance, lifestyle choices, and activity levels. Another accommodation to successfully craft failure-free activities is to accept the fact that they might not always be socially acceptable. The right puzzles for our loved one might be ones normally used by young children or toddlers. One group successfully turned repetitive motions into actions by assembling simple objects. To accommodate a woman who repeatedly made pinching motions in the air, the designer built a rack with clothespins. The woman happily placed the clothespins on the slim bars, took them off, and put them on. We must keep our goal in mind, and set aside norms and traditions to find what keeps our loved one happy and engaged.[269]

Spotlight on Safety—Altering Environments for Safety

By the middle-moderate stages, your loved one may not be able to safely use tools, knives, or scissors; distinguish the white toilet in a light-colored bathroom; safely navigate stairs or steps; or identify items such as shampoo and hand cleaner as being inedible. If your loved one wanders at night, we need to ensure she has a safe place for roaming without getting lost or hurt.

If keeping your loved one safe comes down to changing her behavior or changing her environment, try to find ways to alter the environment first.[270] Remove the knife set from the counter top; hide the candy bars, chips, and deserts; put cleaners such as bleach and ammonia in locked cabinets; put everything she needs on one level to avoid stairs; or make sure sturdy railings are in easy reach of all steps.

If visual perception difficulties make it hard for your loved one to find the toilet in the bathroom, use contrasting colors, blocks or barriers. When Lela Shank's husband, who had Alzheimer's disease, began confusing the tub or sink with the toilet, she cordoned off all but the toilet at night. She also covered the floor vent. With these accommodations, he was able to get up at night and use the bathroom on his own.[271]

Poor lighting, lack of color contrast, clutter, noise, and chaos of the home could be triggering some behaviors. The goal is to reduce anxiety and agitation by altering her environment.[272] Some possible accommodations are: covering mirrors, reducing excess glare or dark shadows, labeling or removing family photographs, reducing noise or clutter, and reducing tripping hazards (such as low furniture or loose throw rugs).[273]

If your loved one is struggling with delusions or hallucinations, TV programming can make it worse because she might have difficulty discerning between fiction and reality. High energy, graphic action adventure shows can fuel delusions and hallucinations or create active dreams.[274] On the other hand, your loved one might do fine with TV, even with the sound off. It all depends on your loved one.

With an impaired ability to discern food from household cleaners and other potential poisons, you will need to restrict access to soap, lotions, candles, floor cleaners, rubbing alcohol, and other solvents, including nail polish remover.[275] During a visit with Mom and my sister Louise, I left them alone to get some oriental take-out at the food court. Since no bathrooms were close by and Mom wanted to wash her hands, Louise handed Mom a small bottle of hand sanitizer. Before she realized what happened, Mom drank the cleanser.

A supportive environment provides clues that can help your loved one find the bathroom or dining room, or point toward the appropriate activities for each area. For example, create defined areas for eating with a well-appointed dining room, or set up an inviting living room with comfortable couches and large windows for socialization. The necessary cues and guides will change with your loved one's progression.[276] Carefully select furniture, decorations, books, clothes, and other items that provide context for the room and her heritage, without overstimulating her. It can help her stay calm and peaceful. Limiting choices can help prevent problems from developing.

In the earlier stages, Mom knew and understood why she wore adult incontinence undergarments. However, she forgot this in the middle stages. She had trouble making it to the bathroom in time due to the combination of slow gait and not being able to find the restroom. Before, she had chosen to put on her adult pads. Now, having forgotten the reason, she began selecting her panties instead. I knew she would not remember repeated instructions or understand notes on what to wear.

In the midst of putting her summer clothes away and pulling out her winter sweaters and heavier pants, I bagged up her panties and filled the drawer with the undergarments. She no longer had to make a choice and she never complained about the missing panties.

Incontinence

If your loved one has trouble remembering where the bathroom is, take her to the bathroom regularly to help reduce accidents. During these stages, my mother usually had no problems once we arrived at the bathroom. Her use of incontinence undergarments was largely precautionary.

However, incontinence can also be triggered by stress, overstimulation, or binge eating. With bvFTD incontinence occurs earlier in the disease and may be triggered by stimulating or stressful environments.[277] If accidents still occur, even while helping your loved one go to the bathroom regularly, and binge eating is under control, look for other causes—stress or anxiety due to noise, commotion, or overcrowding could be the trigger.

Adjusting the Social Environment and Access to Food

Once you have safety-proofed your house and know how to avoid distressing environments, you can also structure meals, meal portions, and time social events to maximize your loved one's social skills.

Your loved one may prefer to eat only particular foods. It's usually not a problem if she wants to eat chicken every day. But if she wants to eat a gallon of ice cream or five candy bars a day, do some planning to avoid weight gain. One family provided small, bite-sized candy bars and hid the bag, satisfying their loved one's craving and reducing her weight gain at the same time.[278] If your loved one is prone to binge eating, keep food out of sight, in a controlled area, and hand out measured servings (don't make the mistake of handing her the bag of chips thinking she will stop when she is full—she might not realize when she has had enough). Put snacks and small meals on a set schedule to control overeating.[279]

Your loved one may no longer recognize she should only eat the food on her plate. If you can't stop her from taking other people's food, you may need to provide supervision when she eats or separate her from others. Also, give her small, healthy snacks throughout the day, or distract her with her favorite activities. One residential care facility installed indoor and outdoor basketball hoops for redirecting the binge eating and food-grabbing behavior of a former basketball player.[280]

Take your loved one out for dinner or to a park when fewer people are present; select calmer, quieter restaurants. If your loved one grows impatient waiting for a meal, plan simpler meals and keep him busy with activities until the food is ready. One caregiver kept her husband busy with walks, large toys, and craft activities. Have things ready to go, and seamlessly move from one activity to the other. It will reduce problems before they occur. The other advantage to keeping your loved one active is he might sleep better at night. The goal is to help your loved one stay content and engaged.[281]

As deficits develop, your loved one may understand written words or pictorial clues better than spoken words. Speech therapists can determine which language modality—reading, writing, listening, or speech—works best for your loved one, along with the most conducive environment. Does your loved one need to be alone in a quiet room to respond? Does he need time to process and react to simple commands, such as 'stand up'? Would flash cards work better? As your loved one declines, you will need to adapt the best methods for communicating.[282]

Sundowning

During late afternoons and throughout the evening, some people with dementia develop increased confusion, agitation, and restlessness. This could be due to fatigue, pain, not enough stimulation during this time of the day, or less light as evening draws nearer. Perhaps overall tiredness from the stress of getting through the day lessens ability to cope at this time.[283]

Check your behavior log for clues to late afternoon and early evening issues. Offer a small snack in the middle of the afternoon to help make it through until supper. Perhaps she needs a dose of pain medication. Taking a short nap or listening to her favorite music while you scurry about getting ready for supper and the evening might be the solution. Try to shelter your loved one from the noise and chaos that naturally develop during these periods.

Conversely, your loved one may need activity and busyness to settle inner agitation. Ask her to help with the preparations, or provide other activities that might distract her. Len Strickler, whose wife had frontotemporal dementia, arranged to keep his wife busy and occupied before supper with activities such as going for a walk or watching TV.[284] For example, if you loved one likes to fold clothes, keep a basket ready to focus her attention.

If you know that your loved one is tired and more easily stressed during this period of the day, plan to do more demanding activities such as bathing earlier in the day.[285] Meet the family at the mall mid-morning and go out to lunch instead of eating supper at a restaurant--schedule events when your loved one is at her best.

Obtaining the Help You Need

You might need to reassess your support network. In the middle stages, the caregiving burden can intensify. Sometimes, it's easy to fall into the trap of thinking you are the only one who can be there for her. Resist the "martyr" complex.

While it might seem counterintuitive to remind yourself to see to your own needs—it's a necessity. If you burn yourself out or become sick, your caregiving will suffer. Providing care for your loved one demands high energy, attention to detail, as well as the ability to react and rotate instantaneously to your loved one's needs. It is critical that you eat properly, keep your emotional balance (as much as possible), and get the rest you need.[286]

Analyze your situation and identify ways you could arrange help so you can get away for a while. Family, friends, and church members are your first line of defense.[287] Sort out those tasks that are best for you to do and identify those other family members or friends can help with. A daughter could take over the more time-consuming financial and tax matters; a son can mow the lawn and help with other household chores; a granddaughter can spend an afternoon sitting with her grandpa so you can go out for coffee. Don't be afraid to ask for specific help, but also guard against getting angry or feeling bitter if they rebuff you. Perhaps God will provide the answer to your need another way.

Adult daycare can give you time each week to get chores done.

Contact your health care providers for facilities that provide respite care or good adult daycare centers. Many people find that having one or two days a week to get things done helps make the caregiving burden bearable. Studies demonstrate that a caregiver needs time away where she can do other things and not focus on the loved one. Lela Shanks, who cared for her husband with Alzheimer's disease, recommended regular respite care should be no less than four hours at a time on a regular basis. She utilized adult daycare as her primary source for caregiving relief.[288]

With adult daycare, your loved one has a safer space for roaming and she is engaged in group activities suited to her abilities. The social interaction is more stimulating than what you can provide at home. She now has a community of peers where she can be a vital part, helping and encouraging others.[289] Utilizing daycare a few days a week may delay entrance into more expensive care facilities.

Many care facilities also provide short-term respite services. They will allow your loved one to stay as a resident on a temporary basis if you need to be away, such as going on vacation or having surgery.

Can friends stay with your loved one while you attend a meeting or support group? In one church, friends sat with the husband so the wife could continue to attend ladies' missionary group meetings. Don't turn away offers, but consider where a helper could lighten your load.

Solutions will vary as you and your loved one move through the stages. While in the earlier stages your loved one might have done fine at home alone for brief periods, or could accompany you on outings or shopping, by the middle stages you might have to find other solutions.

You are blessed to be called to this ministry, but you also must allow others the privilege of serving you. Your calling also represents a calling to friends, neighbors, fellow church members, and others to experience the blessings of helping you. We must never consider ourselves beyond needing help.

So don't be shy about asking for help. Over the years, I learned that God never failed to provide help in times of need. He sometimes used strangers who just happened to be passing by. In moments of need, I cried out to God and He answered.

Accept the help God brings your way. Open your mind to solutions which might not be the ones you anticipated. Perhaps He will work differently this time. Sometimes, He speaks through our loved one. I always kept an ear open for Mom's little pearls of wisdom. One caregiver wracked with guilt about placing her husband in a nursing home was surprised and pleased to hear him say during a rare moment of lucidity that he was fine and he wanted her to be fine, too.[290]

Taking stock, assessing the situation, put one foot in front of the other, looking for ways to work out the obstacles, wrinkles, and bumps. Usually, you can find a solution to make things work. However, be alert for signs you need to create some safe times for yourself free from caregiving responsibilities.

> But he said to me, "My grace is sufficient for you,
> for my power is made perfect in weakness."
> Therefore I will boast all the more gladly of my weaknesses,
> so that the power of Christ may rest upon me.
> 2 Corinthians 12:9

Identify those times and duties in your day which cause the most stress and anxiety. Pray for helpers. People who have known your loved one for a long time might be best suited to visit with him while you shop in the afternoon. Contact social services for paid sitters who can take over during rough periods or give you some time away to refresh yourself. By taking the time you need to recharge, you will make it possible to continue caregiving as well as begin to lay in place future contacts for your life after caregiving.

Use your respite time to push back the isolating burden of being the primary caregiver. Reach out to friends and family, resume past hobbies or interests. In preparation for your loved one's passing, establish relationships with those outside your caregiving circle.[291] Judy Towne Jennings, whose husband had Lewy body dementia, resumed her tennis sessions.[292] Reconnect with your quilting or gardening group; do something not related to dementia. Yes, support groups are invaluable, but you also need to do something different that will help you, for just a brief time, live in a different world.

Burnout

> *Caregivers can get to a point, when one more minute of giving, is too much. Nothing of the self is left except a charred frame ... Specifically, if she can't change things in ways that promote peace of mind while providing care, she needs to remove herself from the caregiving role. And conversely, if there is no other option for the care of the loved one, she needs to make changes in how she is providing care.*[293] Judy Towne Jennings

Caregiving for a loved one can become all-consuming until nothing remains except bearing with her insults, cleaning up the messes, or shadowing her through the night as she wanders. It is easy to not take the time for yourself until you realize you are not sleeping well, bingeing on soda and chips, or barely taking the time to cook complete meals. Everyone needs a break, even caregivers. Not taking the time for yourself can lead to total mental and physical exhaustion, rendering you unable to continue to care for your loved one.[294]

Lack of sleep, poor diet, and never-ending stress can destroy your ability to respond patiently to your loved one. If you find yourself in an emotional meltdown and in a crisis moment, for the safety of yourself and your loved one, you need to get away. Even if you have to hire a sitter, or schedule an extra day at daycare, take time to recharge, reconnect, and refresh. Some care facilities offer respite programs where your loved one can stay for short periods of time. Whatever it takes to get back on track, take the step to withdraw from the burdens of caregiving to recharge.

The stress of burnout can affect your ability to find solutions. If the situation seems hopeless and you feel trapped—no one else can handle him, you can't afford sitters or respite, no one cares enough to help—seek a wise counselor.[295] A godly pastor or close friends, knowledgeable about your situation, can help you find solutions to meet your needs as well as your loved one. Find someone you trust who has a more distant, objective viewpoint. Honestly consider the suggestions—depression, discouragement, and despair can color everything until hopelessness shuts down every option.

Are you feeling overwhelmed, terrified, anxious, or so deeply depressed that getting out of bed takes a herculean effort? Do thoughts of running away or suicide float through your head? Do you find yourself easily irritated and upset with your loved one? Have you hit her, shoved her, or treated her roughly? Did you find yourself walking away, just to get some distance? Are you not sleeping? Are you losing weight or are you craving sweets or caffeine? Do you begin to dread particular parts of the day, such as mealtimes or getting her ready for bed?

If you feel any of these, it's time to get help. To survive providing care to your loved one, you will have to find ways to get your needs met. It is not selfish to take time for things you enjoy when it provides the break and refreshment that will enable you to continue providing for your loved one.

Sometimes as Christians, taught to put God, church, and family first, we find it hard to accept that taking the time we need is not selfishness, it's required. God tells us our bodies are the temple of the Holy Spirit (1 Corinthians 6:19-20). From time to time, Jesus brought His disciples aside for rest and recuperation (Mark 6:31). The Apostle Paul counseled Timothy to take a little wine for his stomach ailments (1 Timothy 5:23).

Jesus tells us that if we take His yoke upon us, it will be light (Matthew 11:28-30). The Bible promises God will supply our needs (Philippians 4:19); that we will have everything we need for life and godliness (2 Peter 1:3).

So why doesn't it feel like this? God promises to not give us burdens we cannot bear. Paul writes, "God is faithful, and he will not let you be tempted beyond your ability, but with the temptation he will also provide the way of escape, that you may be able to endure it" (1 Corinthians 10:13). Why doesn't it feel this way?

God is faithful. If I am struggling, feeling overwhelmed, and at the breaking point, I need to step back and consider:

- Am I trying to do this on my own and not leaning on God for help?
- Have I taken too much for myself, acting as if I were the only one who can take care of Mom, and not willing to delegate some of the responsibilities?
- Am I harboring resentment and anger against God, my loved one, or friends and family who seem to be failing me?
- Am I struggling with extending care to someone with whom I have a bad relationship to begin with? Am I holding onto slights, grudges, and bitterness from the past? Am I giving into thinking they failed me in the past and now they are ruining my life?

Is there a particular time of the day or situation where you have the greatest problem? Analyze what you are thinking and your reactions to your loved one's comments or behaviors. Sometimes, what she says pushes our buttons. We feel unloved, neglected, unappreciated, criticized. Reacting to her as she was before the dementia can cause inner conflict. We have to choose to remember that without the dementia, she would have never said those things.

How do we handle this? We need to remember: "For though we walk in the flesh, we are not waging war according to the flesh. For the weapons of our warfare are not of the flesh but have divine power to destroy strongholds" (2 Corinthians 10:3-4). Our loved one is not the enemy—the ravages of the disease are the enemy; she is its victim.

We need to reframe the conflict and step back. She is still our loved one, but her ability to acknowledge and affirm that has changed. We must now acknowledge and affirm her worth to us by helping her be all she can be. So, we try to let her comments roll off our backs. We seek to find ways to help her live well, day by day.

In the beginning when Judy Towne Jennings' husband was first diagnosed with Lewy body dementia, she tried to bargain with God and asked for a miracle. She realized she needed to express her inner thoughts and bring them to the surface.[296] She found journaling was a way to talk with God and reveal her deep emotions. Her soul was refreshed so she could continue caring for her husband.[297]

If God called us to this ministry, He will enable us to complete it His way. So, we have to ensure we are not taking on more than we should, but willingly delegate. I thought of myself as Mom's advocate, working with the staff at Sienna Crest, checking her medications in consultation with her doctor, and ensuring all her needs were met.

God provided help at the right time. Periodically, my sisters visited and took Mom places. Sienna Crest had activities. My husband was a ready listener as I shared the latest activities and stories about how Mom was doing. I found coworkers or friends at church who listened and gave advice. Often the Sienna Crest staff helped me understand the intent or meaning behind Mom's actions.

Through it all, we can be assured that God will provide just the right means, at the right time, the right services, the right health care workers and facilities, the right helpers, so you, just the right caregiver, can help this child of God walk her last years on earth well.

Hard Decisions in the Middle-Moderate Stages

Surgeries and Hospitalization

Our loved one might have other health issues leading to surgery or hospitalization. These events can be traumatic—hard on the body and the soul—even for healthy people. As mentioned in Chapter 2, this can bring on delirium in the elderly. Contemplating these options for our loved ones with dementia can lead to hard choices.

Investigate all options including a less intrusive procedure that would be just as effective. Do not forget to consider the dementia factor. Your loved one's cognitive difficulties may impact recovery.

Confusion, disorientation, or lack of cooperation could make recovery therapies less effective; the medications required might have harmful side effects, especially if your loved one has Lewy body dementia. Make sure you go over the medications with a physician knowledgeable about prescription drug interactions with your loved one's disease(s).

Beware Surgeries

After surgery, some people develop problems with cognition from which they never fully recover. They continue to have problems with memory, concentration, and confusion. It is not known whether this is primarily due to the effects of the anesthesia, inflammation, the higher concentrations of oxygen delivered during longer surgeries, or the illness itself.[298]

If your loved one develops another condition that might point to surgery, investigate all the options with your medical team. Carefully and prayerfully weigh all the benefits and risks. Your loved one with dementia might not be able to comprehend what will happen during a surgery. She might not understand why she cannot have any food or drink the night before. She might have trouble with the after-surgery therapy and rehabilitation. If her ability to communicate is compromised, it will be difficult to know if her pain is properly controlled. Consider whether the benefits of the treatments outweigh the possibility of further cognitive decline.

Keep Company When in the Hospital

Our loved one does best in a familiar environment with consistent routines and the usual caregivers. As an illness or injury impacts your loved one's cognition at the same time her support system is withdrawn, her ability to cope with the busyness of a hospital is eroded. This can lead to confusion, agitation, and aggression.[299]

Dr. Mary Newport experienced this when her husband Steve, diagnosed with Alzheimer's, was in the hospital. She had originally attributed the decline following hospitalization to the illnesses that cause dementia, but she also discovered hospital standard procedures also contributed to the difficulties. Steve's episodes of confusion were handled with chemical and physical restraints. The enforced bedrest eroded his strength and ability to walk. Dr. Newport attributes much of her husband's decline in the hospital to the hospital staff's lack of understanding concerning the needs of dementia patients, as well as insufficient time to provide adequate care.[300]

Hospitals are geared toward treating cognitively aware patients. Staffing does not permit hospital workers the time to help your loved one with dementia go to the bathroom or eat a meal. Not understanding your loved one's way of communicating, the staff often does not perceive that agitation could signal unmet needs, such as having to go to the bathroom, being hungry, or in pain. Your loved one can rotate from lucidity to confusion in a brief period of time and become resistant to nurses taking vital signs, staff drawing blood for tests, or begin removing tubes and intravenous lines.

Try to have a knowledgeable friend or family member stay with the loved one during her time in the hospital.[301] The familiar caregiver will be able to help your loved one eat, get up to go to the bathroom or walk. A sitter, familiar with your loved one's ways of communicating, can keep her calmer and reduce the need for medications to control behaviors. Remember that being bedbound even for a short time can make anyone weak and unsteady. Ensuring your loved one is getting up to go to the bathroom and moving about will help maintain her strength.

Monitor the medications they give her to ensure her regular medicines are administered, and follow up if the hospital doctors are prescribing drugs not suitable for her. Work with your medical team, and provide a list of drugs that have been shown to be dangerous for your loved one. Be aware of the side effects of these drugs. Try to ensure your loved one's daily dementia medications are administered regularly and at the right times.

Some hospitals will administer Haldol (Haldol is the brand name for haloperidol, an antipsychotic drug) if a patient becomes agitated or disruptive, such as trying to rip out lines and tubes, or resisting treatment. While many hospitals and nursing homes find Haldol effective in controlling disruptive behavior, this drug and others similar to it can produce adverse reactions that might become permanent if the medication is not stopped in time.

These types of typical antipsychotic drugs can cause permanent damage or even bring on death, especially for a loved one with Lewy body dementia. The Food and Drug Administration (FDA) has a black box warning on this drug citing greater risks of stroke and death in elderly patients with dementia.[302]

The signs for adverse reactions to antipsychotics are " …high fever, sweating, unstable blood pressure, stupor, muscular rigidity, and autonomic dysfunction."[303] Some will develop *tardive dyskinesia,* which is sweating; temperature spikes; irregular blood pressure; rigid muscles; or dazed look. This serious reaction to Haldol is recognized by having difficulty swallowing, chewing motions, tongue thrusting, twitches in the face and jaw, tremors, or rolling motions with the fingers. Many of these symptoms are uncontrollable and frequent.[304] In some instances, this drug can be fatal.

Dr. Newport observed some of these symptoms when her husband Steve was in the hospital. Upon investigation, she discovered that when he became confused in the evenings, the staff administered Haldol, even though she alerted the physician to her husband's adverse reactions to it.[305] If your loved one develops these symptoms, research the administered medications and discuss substituting safer therapies or drug alternatives with the attending physician.

A family member, friend, or sitter knowledgeable about your loved one will know how to interpret periods of agitation. They can help make sure she continues to eat and keep her calm so the nurses do not need to administer antipsychotics. Sitters are even more critical if your loved one has Lewy body dementia. Many hospital workers don't understand that she can become confused or lose consciousness without warning, or that she is prone to fainting when standing.

One caregiver left his wife at the hospital to go home to sleep. He explained to the staff that she could not be left alone because she fainted every time she stood up. Despite the warning, his wife was left alone in the room with the bed's guardrails up. The staff did not realize she could crawl around the rails to get to the bathroom. She managed to get to the edge of the bed and stood up without waiting for her blood pressure to stabilize. She fainted when her blood pressure plummeted, and broke her ribs, leading to pneumonia and death within two months.[306]

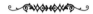

Assume your loved one will require more vigilance and round-the-clock care when in the hospital. Follow up on medications, make sure she gets the ones she needs, and find the help to guide her through her moments of confusion and distress. Perhaps an alternative exists that can be administered in familiar surroundings with caregivers she trusts. Avoid hospitalizations if at all possible.

Do Not Resuscitate Order (DNR)

Cardiopulmonary resuscitation (CPR) was originally developed to revive otherwise healthy patients in a medical emergency. This procedure seeks to restore heartbeat and breathing when a person's heart has stopped. It involves continuous rapid chest compressions, sometimes with rescue breaths, or direct current defibrillation.[307]

How well do people with dementia handle CPR? Dr. Ladislav Volicer's 2005 review of studies for the Alzheimer's Association found CPR was three times more likely to produce negative outcomes in persons with dementia. Even if the patient survived the procedure, most died within twenty-four hours.[308] Age and disease can render the body less fit to absorb the physical damage caused by CPR. The few who do survive never fully recover. It can break ribs, puncture lungs, and lead to infections.[309]

CPR has become standard care provided by emergency and hospital staff. Even if your loved one has stated in her advance directive or living will that she does not want CPR, many states require CPR to be performed if breathing and the heart stop. There is assumed consent to CPR unless a do-not-resuscitate order (DNR) exists.[310]

To avoid your loved one having CPR performed on her in the ambulance or at the hospital requires a DNR from the doctor. This is a medical order written when your loved one is considered terminally ill or too frail to benefit from CPR.

When Lois, the Sienna Crest director, suggested I get a DNR for my mother, Mom could still make some decisions. During an office visit, the doctor presented the realities of CPR and she agreed to the order. If Mom had passed the point where she could make this decision, I could have done it for her as her designated representative in her durable health care power of attorney.

Remember: DNR Does Not Mean Do Not Treat

A DNR is not an order to stop all medical treatments. Your loved one should still be treated for pain, infections, and injuries. As her caregiver, make sure the medical staff continues to treat your loved one just as before the DNR was written, apart from cardiopulmonary resuscitation.

Unfortunately, many doctors do not understand that a DNR order refers only to CPR and not to other treatments. "Misunderstandings among physicians about living wills, advance directives, and do-not-resuscitate orders are common, according to research and medical experts."[311] Insist that your loved one is treated for other medical conditions and her care is not limited. After asking many questions of the Sienna Crest staff and the doctor, I assured my sisters that Mom would still be treated for arising medical needs, such as infections. Once the order was signed, she wore a DNR bracelet to alert medical personnel.

Considering a Residential Facility

Many of us desire to keep our loved one at home in a familiar environment for as long as possible. However, as the disease(s) progress, your loved one might eventually reach a point where home is not the best option. Has he become combative, is he reacting violently to hallucinations, does he need medical care you can't safely provide at home? If he is no longer able to transfer from chair to bed or to stand on his own, can you lift him or keep him from falling without hurting yourself?[312] Is he beginning to wander throughout the night? These developments might make it necessary to find a residential care facility or nursing home for him.

Some caregivers have the health, stamina, and capacity to provide comprehensive care, and can make the changes in the home to provide a safe, nurturing place for the loved one. Many spouses have successfully cared for the loved one with dementia to the end.

Dr. Yasyn Lee, MD, a geriatric psychiatrist in Dubuque, Iowa, said in a presentation that a patient with dementia can remain at home if he remains calm and does not become disruptive. However, once wandering or aggressive behaviors develop, moving to a nursing home should be considered.[313] When your loved one gets up throughout the night, can no longer transfer from bed to wheelchair, or sometimes reacts violently, that is the time to consider other alternatives. These behaviors can put the loved one or his caregiver in danger.

Seeing ourselves as executive management, we have to step away from our emotional attachment and objectively consider the best place for our loved one. Home might or might not provide the optimal care. Nursing homes have professional caregivers on shifts— one caregiver cannot provide round-the-clock care. Staff does not carry the emotional baggage of past slights, feelings of inadequacy, or the disappointment of what has been lost with the disease. They do not perceive the loss of function and accomplishment your loved one has experienced. They are well-suited for taking care of your loved one as he is, not as he had been.[314] It is difficult to admit that our loved one's needs could be met by strangers in a facility. Our loved one might do very well under the care of a professional team—I learned many things when talking with the staff at Sienna Crest.

Our role of caregiver does not stop; the facility does not take over. We do not put our loved one away. Neither do we abandon him to strangers, giving no further thought of his needs. We now work with a team that will enrich and expand the resources available to our loved one. Our intimate knowledge of our loved one's background and history, combined with the staff's knowledge of helping people, optimizes our loved one's care. We now have the time and energy to minister to his needs as close family and friends.

In the book *No Act of Love Is Ever Wasted,* Jane Thibault and Richard Morgan describe a family where the wife, stricken with dementia, thrived in the right nursing home. While her husband at first resisted the idea, once she moved there, she interacted with others more and was less irritated with her husband. His visits with her became congenial. Even though she might not recognize him as her husband, they were able to continue their mutual love and affection despite the changes dementia brought. Her husband found support and friendship through his contacts with the staff and the home's caregiver support group.[315]

Not everyone is suited to perform the duties of daily care—such as bathing or clipping nails. Our loved one might be happier if a trained professional takes on these tasks. Our caregiving now revolves around advocating for her needs and loving her as close family.

Finding the Right Place

Investigate the best facility for your loved one: the best fit will not only accommodate her current needs, but will work with her as she transitions through the stages. You want to prevent transferring your loved one to a different facility as the dementia advances. Many facilities can adjust to increasing cognitive difficulties. Your loved one will not have to bear the additional burden of adjusting to a new place with different routines and caregivers.[316]

There is great variety in facilities, ranging from assisted-living centers to nursing homes. Each area has its own mix with varying names for the options. Work closely with your doctor and medical care providers for suggestions and referrals. Also, consider your loved one's unique temperament—is she gregarious as my mother was, thriving in social environments, or does she prefer greater privacy with less social interaction.

Ensure the facility is able to handle the challenges your loved one brings. Investigate their protocols and procedures for behaviors. Seek out a facility that is willing to work with your loved one's issues. Is the staff trained to handle these problems?

A good center will be willing to work with you in crafting a care plan. You, of course, continue to be the advocate for your loved one, seeing that her needs are met. Drawing from your knowledge of her history, you can be a resource to the facility in crafting care solutions.[317] You still remain the go-to person for helping your loved one get through his day.

Ask a lot of questions; visit facilities at different times of the day; talk with directors, staff, and families of other residents; check out any complaints. Watch how staff interacts with residents—do they treat them as family or more distantly.

Dr. Zeisel specializes in environmental design of facilities to utilize and enhance cognitive capabilities. He recommends that dementia units have: a homelike environment with rooms decorated to fit their purpose, such as dining rooms, living rooms, and activity rooms; camouflaged and secure exits that allow the residents to move freely without feeling trapped; destinations at the end of hallways with landmarks that help residents find their way; safe outdoor spaces with gardens; and places where residents can place familiar objects.[318] Some facilities have shadow boxes near the door to a resident's room where she can place mementos and reminders of her life. Dr. Zeisel's work has focused mainly on designing residences for people with Alzheimer's-type dementia.

Work with the facility to help your loved one adjust to her new home. Don't stop your behavior log. This will help you keep the staff accountable and is a good reference for highlighting changes to care. Share your loved one's past accomplishments and way of life so the staff can interact with her as a person.[319]

Residential Facilities for Frontotemporal Dementia (FTD)

Your loved one may be younger, stronger, and healthier than the average person with Alzheimer's-type dementia. The facility best equipped to provide care to your loved one might not be the one nearest you. The facility should be able to accommodate your loved one's compulsive behaviors, including roaming or frequently searching for food. Many with FTD interact less and participate in fewer group activities.[320]

Be up front about your loved one's challenging behaviors. Inform the staff of your loved one's daily routines so they can follow it as closely as possible. Introduce your loved one to the staff, sharing stories and photos of his life, making it easier for staff to relate to him even when he does not smile or respond to overtures of friendliness.[321]

A good facility for a loved one with FTD is able to develop specialized care for each resident, utilizing behavior techniques, as well as carefully controlled prescription solutions. The wide-ranging behaviors with FTD require a facility to find creative ways to structure schedules; remove dangerous objects, such as knives or scissors, from view; provide feeding stations for roaming residents; limit access to food to control overeating; and vary communication methods depending upon the loved one's capacities. For example, if visual language capabilities are mostly intact, the staff could direct a resident with written instructions, as well as verbal commands.

Residential Facilities for Lewy Body Dementia (LBD)

People with Lewy body dementia require staff knowledgeable about medication issues; understand movement problems and know how to decrease falling; able to assist with swallowing difficulties; and are adequately staffed to deal with the fluctuating cognition, fainting, and other system difficulties.

Making the Decision

The optimal resolution is for the family and your loved one to agree to the decision. We had an easy time when Mom realized Sienna Crest was perfect for her after staying there on a short-term basis. As much as it depends on you, seek to help your loved one understand the wisdom of the decision.

If you talked about this move earlier, remind her of what she had said. However if you meet resistance, ask your doctor for help. Your loved one may more willingly follow the advice of a physician or other authority figure.[322]

Sometimes, as the primary caregiver, you have to make an unpopular decision. Even if you stated your intention to keep your loved one at home in the past, take the step to find the right facility. It fulfills your commitment to ensure your loved one is properly cared for. She may not understand. But, you must remember she does not have the ability to make a truly informed, reasoned decision. With prayer, consultations, and courage, continue seeking the best care for your loved one.

Relocation Stress Syndrome (RSS)

Relocation Stress Syndrome (RSS) refers to the temporary increase in cognitive disorientation, agitation, and difficult behavior due to changes in routine and place of living.[323] This is especially true for your loved one with FTD.

Knowledgeable facilities will engage in careful planning to make the first two-to-four weeks of transition a positive experience. Taking into account your loved one's usual behavior patterns, as well as your emotional distress, the facility will seek to provide a calm non-threatening environment with reduced triggers. After in-depth consultations, work with the facility's care plan and suggestions. They might recommend no visits for a period of time or reduced visits, such as short visits just before meal time.[324]

Be open and honest about your caregiving challenges at home. Make sure the facility agrees with your level of medication and is willing to work with your medical team. Be flexible about care plans the facility develops, but do ask questions for clarification. For example, some facilities will limit television viewing since it can trigger delusions or hallucinations.[325]

The Joys and Sorrows of the Middle-Moderate Stages

While the middle-moderate stages are difficult with declining abilities, coupled with sometimes challenging behavior, there are still many opportunities to connect with your loved one. She remains the same person, yet responds to us differently. We can continue to choose to love her with all our being.

Leaning on the Lord, we continue to make the best use of our time with our loved one (Ephesians 5:16). We have her with us for a little while longer. Let us focus on what remains, not on what's lost; let us dig deeper with God, strengthening our faith; and let us not miss those opportunities God brings our way to share the light of Christ in a dark world in the midst of the dementia journey.

⁂

I saw Mom more on the weekends since workday visits were a little harder to manage. She was in bed by 7 p.m., and I needed to be disciplined enough to leave work so I could visit before supper. This also made it easier to head for home—when it was time for supper I helped her find her seat in the dining room, and sat a little bit before leaving.

Just before I entered Sienna Crest after work, I stilled my soul, calmed my breathing, consciously relaxing, I reached for the door knob. I imagined myself exiting my world and entering hers. I stepped across the threshold, praying I would be able to talk with her and understand what she was trying to say.

Then, I smiled as I began my search for Mom. She could be anywhere, but often she would be sitting on the front couch with some of the other ladies. I found a nearby chair or perched on her walker. We chatted, watched the birds land on the trees, the leaves wiggle with the breeze or the snow fall slowly onto the bushes. We rarely talked of anything of substance, but of the weather, the latest special event (Sienna Crest held little parties throughout the year— my favorite was the Caribbean party in January), or shared highlights of the day. We laughed and smiled.

Sometimes the visit with my mother was the more relaxing part of my day.

---

[230] Shanks, p 63.

[231] Nancy D Pearce, *Inside Alzheimer's: How to Hear and Honor Connections with a Person who has Dementia* (Taylors, SC: Forrason Press, 2007), pp 10-11.

[232] Robertson McQuilkin and Paul Copan, *An Introduction to Biblical Ethics: Walking in the Way of Wisdom, Third Edition* (Downers Grove, IL: IVP Academic, 2014), p 35.

[233] McLay and Young, p 110.

[234] Massimo and Hall in Radin and Radin, pp 250-251.

[235] Len Strickler, "Frontotemporal Dementia (FTD) from a Caregiver – Part 5: Top 3 Things Caregivers Need to Know." Alzheimer's Support Network. https://www.youtube.com/watch?v=Jhwbqz8xpdK. Accessed 8/5/2016.

[236] Massimo and Hall in Radin and Radin, p 251.

[237] Amy P Lustig, PhD, MPH, CCC-SLP, "Chapter 10. Getting It Down and Getting It Out: Swallowing and Communication Concerns," in Gary Radin

and Lisa Radin (eds.), *What If It's Not Alzheimer's?: A Caregiver's Guide to Dementia*, 3rd ed. (Amherst, NY: Prometheus Books, 2014), p 175.

238 Ibid., p 180.

239 Ibid., pp 177-180.

240 Ibid., p 185.

241 Whitworth and Whitworth, p 142.

242 Petersen, p 275.

243 Cummings, p 213.

244 The Association for Frontotemporal Degeneration, "In FTD, Roaming Is Not Wandering," *Partners in FTD Care*: Spring, 2013. www.theaftd.org/wp-content /uploads/2011/09/spring-2013.pdf. Accessed 4/6/2016.

245 Scott Silknitter, Robert D Brennan, RN, NHA, MS, CDP, and Vanessa Emm, BA, AC-BC, ACC/EDU, CDP, *Activities for the Family Caregiver: Frontotemporal Dementia/Frontal Lobe Dementia/Pick's Disease* (Greensboro, NC: R.O.S. Therapy Systems, LLC, 2015), p 13.

246 Bruce L Miller, MD, and Rosalie Gearhart, RN, MS, CS, "Chapter 17. A Balance of Health: Maintaining General Medical-Care Practices," in Gary Radin and Lisa Radin (eds.), *What If It's Not Alzheimer's?: A Caregiver's Guide to Dementia*, 3rd ed. (Amherst, NY: Prometheus Books, 2014), p 276.

247 Towne Jennings, p 32.

248 Whitworth and Whitworth, p 123.

249 Ibid., p 98.

250 Mace and Rabins, p 187.

251 Richard Taylor, Ph.D. *Alzheimer's from the Inside Out* (Baltimore: Health Professions Press, Inc., 2007), pp 59-60.

252 Angelica, pp 14, 17, and 26.

253 McLay and Young, pp 108-109.

254 Zeisel, pp 162-163.

255 McLay and Young, p 81.

256 Silknitter et al, p 50.

257 P Murali Doraiswamy, MD, and Lisa P Gwyther, MSW, with Tina Adler, *The Alzheimer's Action Plan: What You Need to Know—What You Can Do—about Memory Problems, from Prevention to Early Intervention and Care* (New York: St. Martin's Press, 2008), p 228; and Whitworth and Whitworth, p 135.

258 Petersen, p 263.

259 Dr. Yasyn Lee, MD, "Calming the Seas of Dementia: The Role of Psychiatric Medications in Easing Behavior Disturbances," presentation 3/22/2016, at Oak Park Place, Dubuque, Iowa, an integrated retirement community with independent living, memory care, and skilled nursing units.

260 Zeisel, pp 70-71.

[261] List developed from: McLay and Young, p 88; Petersen, p 271; and Zeisel, pp 30, 125-126.

[262] Cummings, p 183.

[263] Ibid., p 199.

[264] Ibid., pp 189-190.

[265] Petersen, p 106.

[266] Silknitter et al., p 21

[267] Cummings, p 262.

[268] Zeisel, p 81.

[269] The Canadian Centre for Health and Safety in Agriculture, "Engaged caregiving and stage-appropriate activity for individuals with frontotemporal dementia." https://www.youtube.com/watch?v=KOgkDE3brkE. Accessed 9/23/2017. Excellent video on creating stage appropriate activities out of everyday objects and common toys. And the Association for Frontotemporal Degeneration, "Think Like an Occupational Therapist: The Importance of Individualized Activities in FTD Care." *Partners in FTD Care* Summer 2016. http://www.theaftd.org/wp-content/uploads/2016/10/PinFTDcare_Newsletter_summer2016.pdf. Accessed 9/23/2017.

[270] Petersen, p 308.

[271] Shanks, p 46.

[272] Lisa Ann Fagan, MS, OTR/L, "Chapter 14. Within These Walls: Creating a Safe and Supportive Environment," in Gary Radin and Lisa Radin (eds.), *What If It's Not Alzheimer's?: A Caregiver's Guide to Dementia*, 3rd ed. (Amherst, NY: Prometheus Books, 2014), p 223.

[273] Ibid., pp 223-225.

[274] Whitworth and Whitworth, p 89.

[275] Petersen, p 316.

[276] Fagan in Radin and Radin, p 228.

[277] The Association for Frontotemporal Degeneration, "It's Complicated! Incontinence Management in FTD." *Partners in FTD Care* Winter, 2014. www.theaftd.org/wp-content/uploads/2011/09/January-2014.pdf. Accessed 4/6/2016.

[278] The Association for Frontotemporal Degeneration, "Emotionally Absent: The Loss of Empathy and Connection in FTD." *Partners in FTD Care*, Fall 2014, 2. www.theaftd.org/wp-contents/uploads/2014/12/PiC-fall-2014.pdf. Accessed 4/6/2016.

[279] The Association for Frontotemporal Degeneration, "Hyperoral Behavior in FTD: Changes in Eating and Managing Related Compulsive Behaviors." *Partners in FTD Care*, Winter 2015, 4. www.theaftd.org/wp-content/uploads/2015/04/PIC-winter-2015.pdf. Accessed 4/6/2016.

[280] Ibid.

281 Deborah Thelwell, "FTD—Aspects and Experiences of Frontotemporal Degeneration: FTD—Ever Decreasing Circles." https://deborahthelwell. wordpress. com/2016/04/18/ftd-ever-decreasing-circles/. Accessed 9/23/2017.

282 The Association for Frontotemporal Degeneration, "Communication Strategies in Frontotemporal Degeneration." *Partners in FTD Care* Winter 2012. www.theaftd. org/wp-content/uploads/2011-09/January-2012.pdf. Accessed 4/6/2016.

283 Mace and Rabins, pp 239-240.

284 Len Strickler, "Frontotemporal Dementia (FTD) from a Caregiver—Part 3: FTD Behaviors." Alzheimer's Support Network. www.youtube.com/watch?v=mFDMp Wu9Kjw. Accessed 9/1/2016.

285 Edyth Ann Knox, "Tips on Sundowning in Alzheimer's Patients." www. healingwell.com/library/alzheimers/knox2.asp. Accessed 9/23/2017.

286 Petersen, p 247.

287 McLay and Young, p 68.

288 Shanks, pp 107, 117.

289 McLay and Young, pp 124, 128.

290 Castleman et al., p 27.

291 Thelwell.

292 Towne Jennings, p 31.

293 Ibid., p 30. Quote used by permission from the author.

294 Petersen, p 247.

295 Mace and Rabins, pp 418-419.

296 Towne Jennings, p 115.

297 Ibid., pp 32-33.

298 Newport, pp 246-247.

299 Mace and Rabins, p 197.

300 Newport, p 162.

301 McLay and Young, p 166.

302 Newport, p 239.

303 National Institute of Neurological Disorders and Stroke, "NINDS Neuroleptic Malignant Syndrome Information Page." www.ninds.nih.gov/disorders/neuroleptic_syndrome/neuroleptic_syndrome.htm. Accessed 9/23/2017.

304 National Institute of Neurological Disorders and Stroke, "NINDS Tardive Dyskinesia Information Page." www.ninds.nih.gov/disorders/tardive/tardive. htm. Accessed 12/8/2016.

305 Newport, p 170.

306 Whitworth and Whitworth, p 213.

307 National Cancer Institute, "CPR." www.cancer.gov/publications/dictionaries/cancer-terms?CdrID=744629. Accessed 12/6/2016.

[308] Ladislaw Volicer, MD, PhD, (2005). "End-of-life Care for People with Dementia in Residential Care Settings." Alzheimer's Association. www.alz. org/documents/ national/endoflifelitreview.pdf. Accessed 12/6/2016.

[309] Comfort Care Choices, "Allowing for Natural Death—Myth & Reality." www.comfortcarechoices.com/index.php?option=com_content&view=arti cle&id=59:allowing-for-natural-death-myth-a-reality&catid=36&Itemid=75 Accessed 8/23/2016.

[310] JL Brerault, MD, ScD, MPH, CIP, (2011). "DNR, DNAR, or AND? Is Language Important?" *Ochsner J* 11(4):302-306. https://www.ncbi.nlm.nih. gov/pubmed/ 22190879. Accessed 9/24/2017.

[311] American Medical News, "Clearing up confusion on advance directives." www.amednews.com/article/2012/029/profession/310299941/4/. Accessed 8/26/2016.

[312] Towne Jennings, p 30.

[313] Dr. Yasyn Lee, MD, "Calming the Seas of Dementia: The Role of Psychiatric Medications in Easing Behavior Disturbances."

[314] Cummings, p 182.

[315] Jane Marie Thibault, PhD, and Richard L Morgan, PhD, *No Act of Love Is Ever Wasted: the Spirituality of Caring for Persons with Dementia* (Nashville, TN: Upper Room Books, 2009), p 65.

[316] McLay and Young, p 153.

[317] Whitworth and Whitworth, p 193.

[318] Zeisel, pp 138-141.

[319] Whitworth and Whitworth, p 194. And The Association for Frontotemporal Degeneration, "Emotionally Absent: The Loss of Empathy and Connection in FTD." Fall 2014.

[320] The Association for Frontotemporal Degeneration, "Easing the Transition: Residential Long-Term Care and FTD." *Partners in FTD Care*, Fall 2015. www.theaftd.org/wp-content/uploads/2015/05/PinFTDcare_Newsletter_Fall 2015.pdf. Accessed 4/6/2016.

[321] The Association for Frontotemporal Degeneration, "Emotionally Absent." Fall 2014.

[322] McLay and Young, p 163.

[323] The Association for Frontotemporal Degeneration, "Easing the Transition." Fall 2015.

[324] Ibid.

[325] Ibid.

7

The Late-Severe Stages

"I felt unlucky because when I was little I didn't quite understand because she was too smart, but when I was older I didn't understand what she was saying when she couldn't talk."
Voices of the Grandchildren — Elizabeth

My mother's halting speech as she tried to recall her words, especially her nouns, turned into brief, terse phrases, sometimes containing only verbs. "I need to go," she would say.

"Where?" I asked.

"I don't know," she replied with that lost, worried look in her eyes.

Over time she lost our names and the understanding of what "granddaughter" meant. She looked at me without understanding the small child in her arms was her latest great-grandson. The grandma the younger grandchildren experienced was different. We had to remember to tell them what she had been like before the dementia.

She did not comprehend when her daughter, Joan, told her she had driven fourteen hours to visit her. Time held little meaning for her as she was led through her day—time to get up, time to go to the dining room, time to rest in the nearest wingback chair. Exhausted by early evening, she was in bed by 7:00, but would often wander the back living room around midnight.

⚜

The busyness, the adventures, and some of the behaviors begin to wane as our loved one moves into the late-severe stages. The safety and security of "home," whether it's your home or a residential facility, becomes her world. Too distressed and confused to handle outings, as well as the encroaching physical difficulties of even getting in and out of the car, make venturing forth too difficult.

Our loved one needs our visits, our attention, and activities suited to her level to keep her as alert and engaged as possible. We need to be observant for late-stage problems, such as having trouble eating; being more likely to fall; outings becoming more stressful and confusing; or having greater difficulty engaging with others. We must adapt to our loved one's changing needs, seeking imaginative solutions. No matter how impaired our loved one's ability to communicate and participate in daily life becomes, we must never forget to care for her with the utmost of concern and respect.

Even as our loved one develops a more masklike face, less able to express love, concern, anger, or impatience, we need to remember she is still with us. We need to maintain the same courtesies we extended to our loved one in the earlier stages: not talking about her in front of her as if she were not there; striving to keep her a part of the conversation; and always being kind, considerate, and compassionate.

Love acts even in the face of smaller and smaller returns. Do all to the glory of God (1 Corinthians 10:31), as service to the Lord. Do not be discouraged by the lack of emotional response or return of affection from your loved one. Endeavor to help your loved one finish her life well. A slight smile, a tender touch on our arm, a meal eaten without choking, another night of sleep, or sitting watching the sunset together becomes our reward.

Considerations for the Late-Severe Stages

The disease(s) will continue to spread throughout the brain: affecting visual and auditory perception, the ability to speak, increasing muscle rigidity and balance problems. These changes make it difficult for our loved one to coordinate what she sees with where she is in the room—resulting in tripping on uneven surfaces, bumping into doors or counters, or falling over low objects. Coordinating muscles and balance when standing, sitting, or trying to transfer from a bed or a car becomes more difficult or happens more slowly. She might lose strength to properly chew her food or lose interest in eating. Our loved one will need increasing help with dressing, eating, finding the bathroom, washing, and brushing teeth.

Perceptual difficulties, along with not being able to process clues of the activity going on around her means she will have increasing difficulty responding to you. It is important we approach slowly from the front and allow her to see what we are presenting to her, as well as giving her the time to respond. If she is startled, she could instinctively strike out to defend herself.[326]

If our loved one is living in a facility and it has been reported to you that she has been "acting out" or hitting, get the facts and investigate thoroughly. Perhaps the staff startled her, causing her to react defensively. Stay on top of any medication changes and insist on changing schedules, altering care, as well as ensuring adequate pain control before agreeing to add or increase antipsychotic medications. These drugs, apart from their danger for those with dementia, can cause daytime drowsiness and increase the likelihood of choking on food, leading to further complications.

Good care at this stage will utilize our loved one's capabilities for as long as possible. My mother had prayed she would always be able to walk, since she nearly lost that ability with her childhood polio. Even with partial paralysis in one leg, she continued to use her walker, even though it took concentrated effort for her to walk around the facility. We made sure she had a wheelchair, but she usually chose to walk. Her assisted-living facility accommodated her requests despite her growing weakness. One day, while accompanying Mom to the dining room for supper, I watched the aide follow Mom with the wheelchair just in case she couldn't make it all the way. That was awesome care. The facility had padded chairs conveniently placed in the longer halls for rest breaks.

Changes to the brain can make it difficult to enjoy food. Sometimes, the ability to taste sweetness remains even as aromas and other taste sensations dim. In the late stages, it is more important to help our loved one ingest calories rather than adhering to a strict diet. Let her eat her favorite foods, even if it's not a balanced diet. She might still be moving or walking through most of her day and will need the added energy.[327]

Be alert for changes to daily care as our loved one's capabilities decrease. As my mother began to lose the strength to chew her food, I requested she be given finely chopped and softer foods. Pay attention to increased levels of confusion, disorientation, or incontinence when bringing her on outings. We came to realize Mom could no longer handle going to full-service restaurants or attending church services. We took her to coffee shops or places such as Panera Bread instead.

As our loved one's ability to process sights and sounds erodes, work with other ways of communicating. Use pictures to represent common needs she might have, such as a glass of water for "thirsty," a plate of food for "hungry," as well as pictures to convey "hello," "goodnight," or "bedtime" can help if she is having increasing difficulty responding to spoken words.

With Alzheimer's-type dementia, memories and skills learned later in life are lost first. If your loved one was bilingual, she might lose her second language and revert to speaking a language you do not understand. Using a picture book and learning some basic phrases might be necessary.[328]

Losing the Ability to Use the Phone, Hearing Aids, or Dentures

Eventually, our loved one may no longer recognize common objects or remember how to use them. She might not remember what it means when a phone rings. This was difficult for my sisters, who had always phoned Mom in the evening. When she picked up the phone and put it in her pocket instead of answering, they knew it was time to use other means. For a while, I placed the calls to my sisters, helping Mom talk with them briefly. They began to send flowers and visited her more frequently.

Problems can arise with hearing aids, glasses, and dentures. Our loved one can forget what the devices are for and what to do with them. If lost, replacement might not be possible. My mother had reached the point where she could not have undergone a hearing test to replace her hearing aids, or endured the discomfort of making molds for new dentures.

I spent a lot of energy keeping track of Mom's hearing aids and dentures when she began to take them out and wrap them in napkins. I knew some of them were inadvertently thrown out. Even if I had thought ahead enough to order two sets instead of one when they had been replaced years ago, she had increasing difficulty remembering what they were for and how to use them.

<hr />

While I accepted that Mom could do just fine without her hearing aids, I was not ready to give up on her dentures. After all, this had been important for my father, and Mom looked so much better with her teeth in.

Sometimes, I had her bottoms, and then her tops, until one day I had both sets. I felt elated. However, Mom was at a hymn sing in the back room so I took the dentures to the aide, asked her to put them in Mom's mouth, and make them stay in after the activity.

When I visited the next day, I was devastated to learn both sets of dentures were missing. Despite days of searching, we never found them. I was distraught at the reality of the loss.

A few days later, I took her to the dining room and helped her sit down. I cut up her food and watched her eat, gumming away as happy as could be. Thankfully, I had requested the softer diet some months before.

I remembered something that happened a few weeks earlier. I had found one set and tried to get her to put them in.

She looked at me as if to say, "What am I supposed to do with these?"

After a few failed attempts to get them seated properly, we walked to her room where I wet them and eventually slid them into place. She was such a good sport, she put up with my efforts, but in the back of my mind I began to realize that her days with dentures were drawing to a close.

The Lord was trying to tell me to let it go. Losing them completely forced me to accept it. In some ways, she looked like an old homeless lady. Acknowledging the inner hurt, I told myself it was okay. She was happy and that was the goal after all.

Her needs shifted and changed. She could hear well enough to get by; she didn't seem to notice she no longer had her teeth. Some days, she even forgot to put on her glasses. I was thankful she never lost those.

One day, I paused just past the front door, scanning the group seated on the couch looking for my mother.

"It's time for supper," Kathy announced. The evening aide at Sienna Crest placed a gentle hand on the nearest lady's shoulder. Four ladies occupied the front couch facing a picture window while others sat in wingback chairs. "Edith," she said as she pulled Mom's walker around with a practiced movement and helped her to her feet.

Mom smiled back, placed her hands on her walker and headed toward the dining area just a few feet away.

I watched the scene play out. My mother's smile was met with Kathy's warm embrace. "You're such a dear," I heard her say to my mother.

The sight of my mother's toothless smile, puzzled eyes, and mussed hair pierced my heart again, yet Kathy was not bothered. Thankfully, the staff had a warm affection for my mother, which I greatly appreciated. It was easier for them to accept her as she was.

What of the pert, outgoing, ambitious woman who overcame partial paralysis from polio to raise a family and eventually become a registered dietician? My father would have been appalled that she managed so well without her teeth. It was almost impossible to keep her hair neat since she no longer took any notice of her appearance.

"I would have to cut her hair tomorrow," I said to myself.

Her favorite soft pink sweater was dotted with stains. It had pockets where she put the cookies she didn't eat or packets of coffee creamer along with a myriad of other objects.

"I should clean those pockets out again," I reminded myself.

Yet the staff lovingly cared for her with grace and dignity. Even though dementia changed her, she was still my mother and a child of God. Sometimes, the shock of seeing her reminded me of what she lost until I sat by her side to help her with her meal. She was still my mom. I still loved her and the person she was—not even dementia can steal a person's humanity.

In some ways, the later stages seemed harder on us. She had forgotten to worry; she lived, for the most part, in the moment. If she did become stressed, it was not for long. She could wander at will at night since staff was always about to keep her company.

Watch Valuables, Including Wedding Rings

Mom's wedding ring was stolen during the last week of her life. When Mom entered Sienna Crest, Lois, the director, told us to not have valuables or money unsecured. Some months before, I had tried to take the ring to get it cleaned. Realizing Mom could not understand I would only be taking it for a short time, I decided to let her keep it. She treasured the ring and grew distressed when anyone touched it. That was good enough for us. We gave the theft to the Lord since the ring symbolized so much to my mother. We understood she needed to keep it despite the risk.

However if your loved one has an heirloom which she intends to pass on to the family, have the discussion about who should store family valuables or wedding rings. You might choose to let her keep the item as a treasured object of love, safety, and security.

Cueing and Mirroring

During earlier stages, it was sufficient to lay items out in order. This might not be enough anymore. As the dementia progresses, she might have forgotten what to do with them. For example, when she cannot initiate brushing her teeth on her own, put the toothpaste on the toothbrush and help her bring it to her mouth.

If this no longer works, take another toothbrush and do the same to your teeth. Your loved one will most likely mirror your actions and begin to brush her teeth. For a while, once the behavior is started, she can continue with some guidance. Eventually, you might have to do it for her.

To cue for eating, separate the food on her plate in easily accessible piles. Help guide her spoon to scoop up the food. You might have to start with loading the spoon and handing it to her. Try to let her do as much as she can on her own. Eating a meal with her also helps.[329]

The unique mix of your loved one's diseases could mean abilities might still come and go. One day she needs help eating, the next she does more on her own. The goal remains to let your loved one do as much as possible each day. Only increase the help as you see she needs it.

Your Loved One Wants to Go Home

"I want to go home," Mom said anxiously.

"Which home?" I asked.

"I don't know," she replied. Her sentences could be disjointed, and not related to anything. She talked about the man who went upstairs.

Since she lived in a one-story building, I didn't know how to relate. I just listened.

When asked about Mom's insistence on going home, Lois told me, "That is what they say when they begin to fail."

Mom was failing. She was now at the highest level of care. She could barely tolerate any outing, did not understand what the time of day meant. The aides would get her up, help her dress, walk her to the dining room for each meal, and give her a chance to participate in activities. I was at a loss in how to handle her requests to go home.

Sharing my concerns with friends at work, one coworker told me the story of a man who took his wife for a car ride around the block when she grew agitated and insisted on going home.

At first I rejected the idea outright. In my mind, you drove a car to go somewhere to do something. One had to have a destination in mind with a planned activity as the focus of the trip. To see the journey, itself, as the activity was a new concept. It seemed wrong.

Yet, I decided to give it a try. After all, she might not notice or remember that we were just driving in big circles.

That fall, the days were warm and bright and dry. The leaves were brilliant yellows, soft oranges and vibrant reds in the autumn sunlight. Entering Sienna Crest after work that day, I walked up to Mom sitting on the love seat facing the front door. I leaned close to her ear and said, "You want to get out of here?"

A broad smile spread across her face. "Yes," she said with that glint in her eye I had not seen for a while.

After telling the staff what I was up to, and switching out Mom's walker, we made our way to the car at Mom's now standard glacial pace. I set a small stool by the passenger seat and helped her in. We drove around the side streets of our small town, stopping briefly to watch some kids play soccer in a schoolyard. Mom remarked about the trim on the houses, their flower gardens and the colors of the fall leaves. As we turned down the road to Sienna Crest, Mom recognized the street and Sienna Crest in the distance. She began to talk about where she was, where she used to drive, and her favorite stores.

It was such a success that I drove her most afternoons for several weeks. But as the days passed, she began to notice the children less. She sat still, staring straight ahead. Her comments about the neighborhoods or farms we drove by dwindled. As her world shrank yet again, I began to feel these rides were also drawing to a close.

The bright October days merged into November with cooler, shorter days. She had greater difficulty getting into the car. She would freeze midway between her walker and the lower seat in the car, forget how to turn sideways in the seat, and struggled to stand up. One day, she did not make it and I barely managed to get her off the floor of the car. I eventually helped her into the seat, but it felt like this would be her last car ride.

The next day was gray with low clouds and mist in the air. Chilled as I got out of my car, I knew Mom would not like the damp cold. Stepping through the front door, I decided to ask her. I sat by her on the love seat and leaned close. "You know, it's pretty nasty outside right now. How about we walk in here today?"

She agreed, and we began our next set of afternoon adventures— walking around the facility, greeting every resident we met, sometimes helping them work on a puzzle in the back room. If there were no puzzles going, we sat on the back couch until it was time to head to the dining room.

<hr/>

The drives and the walks helped Mom through her times of wanting to go home, along with hugs, listening to her, holding her close, and sitting beside her. I didn't need to tell her she was home—I made that mistake at first. I didn't need to argue with her or point out that no one we knew lived in the city any more—everyone had moved away.

When your loved one says she wants to go home, she needs love and reassurance. If she's adventurous, she might enjoy a ride around the block or a walk around the facility. If she's more solitary, just holding her hand and hugging her might be enough. Be there for her, let her talk, even if she's not making a lot of sense, and try to match her mood.

Still Treat for Pain

As your loved one's ability to communicate decreases, her inner awareness of pain also erodes. Your loved one could be signaling she is in pain with her facial gestures, how she walks, or her resistance to dressing or bathing even while denying her pain. Make sure your loved one is still receiving medication for arthritis, old injuries or other ailments. Your loved one is probably still in pain even if she is not consciously aware of it.[330]

Visiting

Despite her confusion, Mom always greeted me with a broad smile, saying, "I'm so glad you're here."

Some days, she could walk a little bit. Other days, I sat close, held her hand, hugged her, and listened to the few words she could put together.

Often, she looked at me and asked, "Did I marry? Did I have children?" This occurred even though she had greeted me as if she knew me.

In one sense, she had forgotten my name and could not explain how I was related to her; but I believe, in other ways, she did know me.

With a broad smile and some tears in my eyes, I would pat her hand, hug her, and reply, "Yes, Mom. You were married, had four daughters, and I'm one of your daughters. You were a great mom."

She nodded and smiled with relief in her eyes.

There is great value in visiting our loved one, even if she does not remember who we are. We know her history and what she accomplished. We honor God, her, and her memories by remembering for her, by treating her as the close family she is even if she has forgotten on a certain level.

Music Therapy

I remember my mother telling me that hearing is the last sense to go. "If someone is in a coma, we need to talk to her," she said.

Many people with late-stage dementia seem to come to life while hearing music from their past. Research has shown music therapies can reduce agitation and apathy, improve mood, and help your loved one interact more.[331]

Dan Cohen started the nonprofit, MUSIC & MEMORY[SM], to provide individualized music for dementia patients in residential facilities. They load familiar music from the person's past into a player with headphones.

When Wisconsin nursing homes began using this program, use of psychotropic drugs decreased.[332] People who had been nearly catatonic would sing and begin to interact. The amazing transformations have been detailed in a documentary, *Alive Inside*.[333]

While the goal is to find music your loved one enjoyed as a young adult, many people who became Christians later also do well with favorite hymns and gospel songs. Up to the end, Mom continued to go to the Sunday morning hymn sing at Sienna Crest. She also enjoyed the many musicians who came in to play at the facility.

⌒⦁✕✕⟡✕⟡✕✕⦁⌒

One facility found that music therapy with headphones helped some residents regain their ability to participate in other activities. One resident, who had stopped doing the art therapy, sat down, drew a picture and described it while listening to her music.[334]

Activating the Health Care Power of Attorney (POA)

The living will, along with the health care POA your loved one had drawn up earlier, declares general wishes about possible future medical decisions. However, for the designated representative to make medical decisions on a person's behalf requires the activation of the power of attorney. This means having your loved one declared mentally incompetent and unable to make healthcare decisions.

The process for declaring incompetence is controlled by state law and often described in the POA document.

❧━∽✠∿✠∿━❧

One day, Lois invited me into her office and told me it was time to activate my mother's health care power of attorney (POA). Even if a designated POA for medical issues has been selected, the POA cannot make any decisions for the loved one until she has been declared mentally incompetent.[335]

On the advice of the director, I contacted Mom's doctor and he issued the order. Later that week, I read the form. While I intellectually knew the degree of her dementia, seeing it laid out in black-and-white drove home the reality of my responsibility—decisions concerning her life now rested on my shoulders. Even though I still discussed major decisions with my sisters, I had the final say.

❧━∽✠∿✠∿━❧

The living will, along with the health care POA your loved one had drawn up earlier, declares general wishes about possible future medical decisions. However, as noted earlier with the DNR, this often does not translate well in the ambulance, emergency room, hospital or at your loved one's facility.

Physicians Orders for Life-Sustaining Treatment (POLST)

Activating the health care POA when your loved one can no longer make medical decisions gives you the opportunity to see her wishes enforced. However, local and state laws might dictate other measures. Some states have developed more extensive doctor's orders concerning treatment options for chronically or terminally ill people when death within a year might be likely.

Called Physicians Orders for Life Sustaining Treatment or POLST, it has varying names in different states: such as POST, IPOST,

211

MOLST, or COLST. This form contains three sections and provides various options to choose from for selecting when cardiopulmonary resuscitation (the DNR section) would be administered; the level of medical intervention, ranging from comfort care only to full treatment including intubation; and use of feeding tubes. Printed on colored paper that stands out in a patient's file, this form is supposed to go with the patient, be used in conjunction with her advance directives, and be updated as her medical condition changes. This form is designed to be used for patients likely to die within a year.

However, residential facilities in some regions require a signed POLST upon admission. Some states' laws concerning the POLST indicate it cannot be changed if it was written before the activation of the health care POA. Discuss these issues with an elder law attorney or social worker knowledgeable about the POLST laws for your state to determine the optimal timing or necessity for this form.[336]

These orders attempt to translate your loved one's wishes into medical orders—making it more likely they will be followed. Most state laws allow it to be updated. If your loved one's condition changes, revisit the selections to make sure they still apply.

As with the DNR, ensure your loved one's medical needs are still being met. The POLST should not be allowed to be seen as another order not to treat.

One of the POLST selections concerns tube feeding for your loved one. Developing difficulties chewing and swallowing can lead to aspiration or even pneumonia, along with weight loss. However, research has not shown that tube feeding provides any benefit or prolongs life in dementia patients. It does not prevent aspiration pneumonia.[337]

If your loved one is having difficulty with chewing or swallowing, request a speech therapist to develop remedies. Better outcomes resulted from properly prepared foods in limited quantities throughout the day, with your loved one sitting upright, and handfed, if necessary. The patients were found to be happier, more socially engaged, and lived just as long as those with tube feeding.[338] This topic is discussed in greater detail in Chapter 6: The Middle-Moderate Stages in the Frontotemporal Dementia (FTD) Characteristics section.

Choosing the Level of Treatment
Your Loved One Needs

When a loved one experiences a sudden injury or illness, we might need to make a hard choice between aggressive treatment and comfort care. *Comfort care* focuses on relieving pain and suffering during the final stages of a terminal disease. It means selecting treatments that will provide comfort while not initiating therapies with little benefit for your loved one. Comfort care searches for a balanced path between imposing painful, harmful treatments on your loved one that only delay the inevitable and recognizing therapies that ease pain or discomfort. Patients choosing this approach frequently are more comfortable and in less pain.[339]

Each situation is unique with its own parameters and solutions. To find the best solution for our loved one we seek out the counsel of many. What do the doctors and medical teams say? What does the family think, taking into account their knowledge of the loved one's situation? Cry out to God for mercy, grace, and wisdom to know how to proceed. Wait for His answer. Lean on Him at this time. God is faithful to provide the wisdom.

We can only do the best we can with the knowledge we have at the time. Sometimes, we have to stand against the desire of other members of the family who are not close enough to the situation to understand your loved one's prognosis and ability to survive invasive treatments.

We should not second-guess our choices or become sidetracked with guilt if the treatments turn out badly. The doctors said it would help; they really thought she could recover if placed on dialysis. We can treat, but in the end, God determines the life span of our loved one. Whether it's another year or just one more week, that rests with Him.

Eventually, you will realize the end is drawing near. Once the body begins to shut down, we need to understand our loved one is not going to get better. That major procedure or operation won't turn back the oncoming tide of death. At this point, with increasing frailty, she might not survive any operation or intrusive medical treatments. She is not going to rebound or regain lost abilities. We could choose comfort care instead of aggressive treatments. Certainly, if there is a good chance some intervention would improve health, reduce pain, and ease suffering, it should be done.

Despite the differences between the varying diseases which cause dementia, most patients drawing closer to the end stage will sleep more and begin to lose weight, even if eating well.[340] Your loved one may still be walking; if she has frontotemporal dementia, she might still roam most of the time. The fluctuations common with Lewy body dementia means your loved one may still have lucid periods. This makes it hard to discern how advanced her dementia is

Recognizing our loved one is approaching the end, wanting to squeeze the best possible life for her out of her remaining days, we seek to find treatments that make her comfortable. Instead of pursuing treatments of questionable help, rotate to comfort care focused on reducing suffering.[341]

The options for comfort care are *hospice* or *palliative care*. Hospice, paid for by Medicare or Medicaid, utilizes a team of medical professionals to provide holistic comfort care for someone not expected to live more than six months. The team directs care in the loved one's residence, whether in a home or a facility. Some hospice organizations have their own skilled nursing facility.

Palliative care is also comfort care using the team approach, but each service is billed separately. It does not require the assessment that death is about six months away.

Hospice Care

If a condition emerges for which the treatment would be too intensive or intrusive, the comfort care provided by hospice often remains the best choice. Mom had gone past the point where she understood the podiatrist was trimming the corns on her foot so they would hurt less. She was past the point where she could handle office visits. How could she handle a hospital?

You now have a team of doctors, nurses, chaplains, social workers, and trained volunteers at your side to advise and answer questions. Your loved one receives focused attention. The hospice team approach, with weekly visits from nurses, social workers, and volunteers, helps to treat the whole person.[342]

My mother's hospice team found some issues we had overlooked. The attention can help a loved one rebound to some extent. As long as your loved one still qualifies, she could be under hospice care for a while. My mom had the benefit of hospice for eleven months.

Nursing administrator Jan Zimmerman likes to enroll her dementia patients in hospice as early as possible to give the loved one and family time to develop trust and a relationship that feels more like a friend helping than a medical team.[343]

The Medicare criteria for hospice are based on the usual course of Alzheimer's-type dementias. However, the differences for frontotemporal dementia (FTD) patients mean they often do not qualify until a few weeks before the end of life, missing out on the benefits of hospice.[344] With FTD and Lewy body dementia, it is difficult to pinpoint when your loved one might be in his last six months of life. If your loved one does not qualify for hospice, you can try to find a local palliative care program.

⸺◈✖◈✖◈⸺

Eventually, I had to accept my mother's functionality would not stabilize. Muscle weakness, slurred speech, greater difficulties moving, losing abilities to read and write—inch by inch, week by week, she shrank before my eyes. How low could she go?

One day, I received a call from Sienna Crest telling me Mom was on her way to the emergency room (ER). The staff found her collapsed on the floor of her room.

As I drove to meet her at the hospital, I prayed, trying not to give into panic, wondering yet again if this was it. Was the end near?

At the ER, I found Mom confused and deeply frightened. Once I sat on a stool beside her, she grasped my hand with all the strength she could muster. First, I calmed and reassured her. Second, I began to field all the questions the nurses had been asking my mother. After talking with the nurse, I later had a chance to talk with a doctor.

In the end, the medical team could not find any immediate cause and offered no treatments. Once they determined she did not suffer a heart attack or stroke, I brought her back to Sienna Crest.

A few days later, I sat with Lois, trying to find a way to keep my mother from having to endure trips to the ER every time she fell. Lois stated, "By law, if she falls, we have to call the ambulance."

"There's nothing we can do about that?"

"Not unless she's enrolled in hospice."

"How does that help?"

"If she falls, we call hospice instead, and they come here. We do not have to send her anywhere."

After hearing a brief description of how hospice worked, I nodded. I felt encouraged, knowing hospice would work with Sienna Crest's staff. Mom would not have to move to a new facility or endure trips to ER. "I'll talk this over with my sisters and get back to you. How soon could you get her enrolled in hospice?"

Lois smiled and said, "They just have to evaluate her, but I'm sure she meets the criteria."

Describing the incident with my sisters, they all agreed, and Mom was accepted by hospice within a few weeks. I prayed every day she would not fall again until she was officially under hospice care. She did not need another trip to the ER.

Palliative Care

When hospice is not available, but comfort care has become the main focus of your caregiving, palliative care might be a good option. Palliative care still allows for any needed medical treatments—it is not a decision to suspend beneficial therapies. It does not require a doctor to predict death is likely and can be requested once your loved one has been diagnosed with a terminal illness.[345]

Palliative care follows a team approach similar to hospice, working through your loved one's primary care physician or facility. They can provide guidance and referrals for helpful therapies. For example, the palliative care team can find therapists to help with eating and swallowing problems, or to develop alternative ways to communicate. It helps craft treatments that meet current needs without burdening your loved one with unnecessary procedures.[346] However, not funded directly by Medicaid or Medicare, the services will be billed separately.

Working in conjunction with the family, a plan is developed to provide optimal care in the loved one's preferred setting, including the home. The collaboration allows for utilization of resources at hand. Start with your primary doctor or social worker for options available in your area. You do not have to wait until your doctor thinks your loved one is in her last six months of life.

Approaching the End

"So we do not lose heart. Though our outer self is wasting away, our inner self is being renewed day by day. For this light momentary affliction is preparing for us an eternal weight of glory beyond all comparison, as we look not to the things that are seen but to the things that are unseen. For the things that are seen are transient, but the things that are unseen are eternal."
2 Corinthians 4:16-18

The longer periods of sleep and weight loss accelerate as the end approaches.[347] The body begins to shut down. With the diseases that cause dementia, it can seem to happen in slow motion, with a slow, insidious wasting away until only deep eyes, parchment like skin, and sharp bones remain.

Fears about the difficulties during the end stages are common. Can we keep her from suffering too much? Will I be able to handle watching her die? How can I help her when dealing with my own grief? What about the difficult decisions? Who would help? Who would get in the way?

Our loved one is pulling away. We see her disengaging from the cares and concerns of this life bit by bit. Even as we spend time with her, it seems a widening chasm is pulling her away from us. In the Lord, we can have peace; in the midst of the sorrows, we still have the joy of the Lord. This is only for a period of time. We release her to heaven and the full healing she will experience there.

With this in mind, we search for what she still needs; we seek out activities and functions she can still do. Instead of participating in bingo, she sits nearby with her cup of coffee. This now is the extent of her actions. Maybe music therapy awakens her for a little while, but you perceive the specter of death drawing closer.

We can trust God to be with us no matter how it works out—whether a sudden illness, death during sleep, or a more drawn-out process. It took my mother three weeks to go through this process, but God gave us hints the time was drawing closer a few weeks before.

⁓◦⟨✴⟩◦⟨✴⟩◦⟨✴⟩◦⟩⁓

While walking up the main hall of Sienna Crest after work one day, on the lookout for where she could be, I met Jodie, the lead night aide.

She asked, "Was Glenn your father?"

I said, "Yes, he was. How did you know?" Just the week before Mom had again asked me if she had married and had children. If I had asked her the name of her husband, she would not have known it.

"Well, last night around midnight, I found her walking in the back living room. She told me Glenn had been to see her. He told her he would be coming for her soon."

My heart raced with excitement. "Yes, that would be my father. He died six years ago." The end was near. God would come for Mom soon.

Not knowing what to expect, I found her dozing lightly in the back living room. However, she did not look much different than she had the day before. Later that night, I called my sisters and relayed the story.

Sharing stories after Mom's death, I also learned she had been visited by Glenn and the boys a few other times. "The boys?" I asked my sister.

"Remember she had two miscarriages. Those were her boys."

"Oh," I said, pondering what I had also heard from another aide. Mom had told her Anna had stopped by one night. That would have been her aunt who had raised her after her mother died.

After she had the nighttime visitors, her days did not change. A few weeks passed and I began to wonder how long she would exist in this in-between state.

I became more faithful in my visits; more careful of her needs, closely questioning the staff and talking over options with Lois when I felt things needed to change. Overall, they provided wonderful care.

The Active Dying Stage

One Sunday afternoon in late October, I told my husband, Ralph, I would be visiting Mom for an hour or so. That was my plan.

After a thorough search I realized Mom was still in bed and Tammy, the aide, was sitting in Mom's padded chair.

"I can't get this woman to do anything!" she stated. Energetic, outgoing Tammy usually managed to get the residents up and moving.

"That's okay, Tammy." I looked at Mom and she seemed a little tired, but still okay. "I've got this. I'll take care of it."

I sat by her side and held her hand. "Hi, Mom," I called as she seemed distracted. "It's time to get up. You've been sleeping a while."

She worked at focusing on me only to look up at the far right corner of the ceiling. A rapturous smile spread across her face.

I looked over my shoulder and saw nothing. Although I physically could not see or hear what she was seeing, my heart leapt within me. I knew she was seeing glimpses of heaven. The time had finally come. I called Ralph to tell him I was staying. He brought subs and we visited with Mom for hours.

⁂

Mom advanced to the active dying stage when organ systems gradually shut down, including the digestive system, which begins losing the ability to digest food effectively. This explains the loss of interest in food. Mom would eat a few bites of her favorite pudding. We brought her caramel lattes she didn't finish. Her body conserved energy as she barely moved out of bed.[348] To force food or fluids into her system at this time would have been cruel.

Offer, but don't push. Understand that she might only eat or sip small quantities: soft, cool foods like pudding are better than hot, solid, or spicy foods.[349]

Hospice had given me a book detailing the dying process. I shared the information with my sisters, explaining that as Mom's body shut down she no longer needed to eat or drink as she had before. It was a natural process. As the body shuts down, it cannot handle the additional fluid from IV's. The extra fluid causes bloating and builds up in the lungs and can make your loved one feel like she is drowning. When dehydration is part of the natural dying process, the loved one weakens, goes to sleep, and peacefully draws her last breath.[350]

Listen for a change in breathing pattern. Elevating the upper body sometimes eases breathing, but make sure her neck is not bent, driving her chin into her chest.[351] Hospice brought in a hospital bed for Mom once she reached this stage. I bought Mom a full-size body pillow she could hug, or to prop up against her back for support. I also gave her a large, soft stuffed dog. While she had regular pillows to place between her knees, I felt she might appreciate a stuffed animal to hug close to her chest.

During this time, the body conserves energy by concentrating the blood to the vital organs while restricting the flow to the nose, arms, and legs. These parts begin cooling and the skin might become discolored with purple or blue marks or splotches called *mottling*. It usually starts at the toes and works up the legs.[352]

The hospice team had given me the option of prescribing a medication for my mother that would decrease gurgling sounds sometimes heard during this phase. After learning the medicine would not help my mother in any way, but was only administered to make the family feel better, I declined it. "It's okay," I said. "We can handle this."

Despite the gurgling sounds, suction is not a good solution since it is uncomfortable and can increase the mucus. It's best to elevate the upper body.[353]

The nurse also explained that low-dose morphine, administered sublingually in her mouth, would help ease her breathing. They also provided swabs with which we could moisten Mom's lips and mouth during her last days.

⸺✵✵✵⸺

Sidebar: No Shortcuts

The goal to help our loved one finish well includes allowing her to live out her full life.[354]

We are created in the image of God (Genesis 1:27). As the life-giver, He sets the limits of our lifespan—and that of our loved one (Ecclesiastes 3:2).

We honor God's will by rotating to comfort care (care that eases suffering) when the loved one has transitioned to the active dying process. When it is clear the body can no longer heal itself, it is time to focus on care and treatments that reduce suffering—bypassing procedures that would prolong pain.

We help our loved one through the dying process, but we do not hasten it—that's God's call.

The sorrows of this life are pathways to eternity. It's not about us and it's not about this earthly life. It's about walking the paths God sets for our loved one to reveal His glory.

"Rabbi, who sinned, this man or his parents that he was born blind?" the disciples asked Jesus in John 9:2.

Christ answered, "It was not that this man sinned, or his parents, but that the works of God might be displayed in him" (John 9:3).

He encourages the listeners to "work the works of him who sent me while it is day" (John 9:4). Accepting the path set before us, taking the cross placed before us, completing the tasks given to us, we become part of God's work on earth by helping our loved one finish well.

God uses the sufferings of the loved one and the caregiver to mold and shape us into the image of Christ (Romans 8:29). He is preparing us for the next step, the glories of heaven. "For I consider that the sufferings of this present time are not worth comparing with the glory that is to be revealed to us" (Romans 8:18).

Take courage. We do not choose the shortcut of ending the life of the loved one before Christ comes for her.

I imagined Mom would last a few days, maybe a week, but I was mistaken. It took three weeks, but during that time every daughter and all her grandchildren and great-grandchildren had a chance to say goodbye. Her ability to talk was partially restored. We communicated as we had not been able to in the past year.

Most of all, we did not want her dying alone. I made sure someone was with her, and at the end, we kept a vigil during her last few days until one night she slipped away peacefully.

I still kept up my advocacy for her needs. When the protocol for turning her in bed regularly began to cause real agony with her weight loss and stiffer muscles, I called a meeting to see what changes could be made to decrease the pain. They worked out a plan to turn her less, but still enough to avoid bedsores.

During the last few days, her muscles became rigid. She was curled up in a ball and her legs and arms were stiff. The aides massaged her muscles until they could move her. I increased my prayers that the Lord would take her soon.

We told her it was okay to pass on to heaven.

Be thankful if the Lord grants you a chance to say goodbye. Utilize the time to seek forgiveness or release your loved one from past wrongs if accounts have not been settled. Reminisce about his life and accomplishments. Share what is on your heart and mind, for the time is growing short. It's okay to cry.

The Lord is gracious and merciful, giving us just what we need when we need it. Each person's passing to heaven is a unique journey. One woman explained that her husband with dementia was mute for the last year of his life. He did not regain his speech or have a chance to tell his wife goodbye or say he loved her. Secure in her faith and surrounded by loving family and church friends, she was content knowing her life mate was safe in heaven. Other caregivers, at the end, heard their loved ones express their thankfulness for the loving care they received.[355] God is faithful and provides for our needs.

Halfway into the period of the three weeks, I went home and pulled out the file—the one containing her will, cemetery plot deed, her prepaid funeral plan, and a small slip of paper listing the hymns for her memorial service. Seeing her beautiful handwriting, I laid down the note on the desk and had a good cry. It had been some time since Mom had been able to write in her flowing script. Her handwriting reminded me she was going to a place where she would be completely healed—no longer paralyzed, needing glasses, or worrying.

Preplanning done in the earlier stages continued to be a blessing. Her willingness and courage to communicate her memorial preferences helped the whole family. She died in Wisconsin while my father died in New York State. When family asked us why we did not fly her body back to be buried next to her husband, we could answer with assurance, "These were her wishes." So certain that she would be with her Glenn in heaven, she chose to be buried near where she died.

The Joys and Sorrows of the Last-Final Stages

For I am sure that neither death nor life, nor angels nor rulers,
nor things present nor things to come, nor powers, nor height
nor depth, nor anything else in all creation, will be able to
separate us from the love of God in Christ Jesus our Lord.
Romans 8:38-39

Helping our loved one pass on to heaven is a time of joy mixed with sorrow; deep sadness and grief churning with breathless anticipation of our loved one's heavenly homecoming. Imagining her spirit rising on eagle's wings as she was ushered into heaven, I drew from inner wells of hope and joy. The assurance of our faith sustains us; the Spirit upholds us as we step through each moment, hour, and day helping our loved one finish well.

Each loved one has her own unique journey. While we may try to peer ahead, we never really know how it will all happen until it does. Is this the day? Is this the way she will go—pneumonia, or some other way? Whatever twists and turns our loved one experiences through her final course, for any who know Jesus, His is the first face she will see when she passes over.

The joys and little blessings God sends our way differ for all of us. For some, the loved one rallies near the end, able to share his love and appreciation to you. For others, our faith fills in the shadows with the knowledge his love never wavered, even if he can no longer say it.

Holding lightly to our loved one, we release him to the care of the eternal Father. While we strive to ease the physical pain he endures during this stage, we inwardly anticipate his heavenly graduation. No more pain, no more sorrow, the anguishes of this earthly life cast away as he embraces his eternal future.

Sorrow and joy; grief mixed with happiness. We completed the task set before us—we helped our loved one finish well. As God carried us in His sustaining grace, He used us to carry our loved one through her final journey. How we traveled the path is as important as the destination.

Letting go, little by little, we cut the chords that held our loved one to us. Hospice comes for the hospital bed; we clean out her room in the facility; we step through the funeral and memorial process.

The funeral director kept asking if my sisters and I were up to singing, and playing the flute and piano for her memorial service. "Yes," we told him, "we could do it." Calm and at peace, knowing where Mom was at that very moment—dancing and singing with her Savior and Glenn, whole and complete as never before—we stepped through the honoring of her life and giving thanks to our Savior.

Now, we can reach out to our next calling. For if we still draw breath, if we have not yet been called to walk our final paths, there are other jobs waiting for us to do. We can turn again to hopes and dreams that might have been put on the shelf—looking, praying, and considering our future. We begin with doing the next thing.

Even with our assurance of heaven, grief is still an earthly reality. It's okay to feel relief; it's okay to feel the pain of separation and loss. This is how God made us. We are accustomed to the rhythms of our days with our loved ones. It takes time for our souls to let go. Working through grief is one of our next tasks.

Day by day, week by week we continue on. Let us walk our path with God while we wait for our turn when He will come for us. May we have no regrets, not shirking the burdens Christ sets before us.

And I heard a loud voice from the throne saying, "Behold, the dwelling place of God is with man. He will dwell with them, and they will be his people, and God himself will be with them as their God. He will wipe away every tear from their eyes, and death shall be no more, neither shall there be mourning, nor crying, nor pain anymore, for the former things have passed away."
Revelation 21:3-4

326 Cummings, p 151.

327 Ibid., p 157.

328 Ibid, p 197.

329 McLay and Young, p 99.

330 The Association for Frontotemporal Degeneration, "FTD Symptom or Pain—How Can You Tell?" *Partners in FTD Care*, Summer, 2013. www.theaftd.org/wp-content/uploads/2011/09/summer-2013.pdf. Accessed 4/6/2016.

331 CY Cheong, JA Tan, YL Foong, HM Koh, DZ Chen, JJ Tan, CJ Ng, and P Yap, (2016) "Creative Music Therapy in an Acute Care Setting for Older Patients with Delirium and Dementia." *Dementia and Geriatric Cognitive Disorders Extra* 6(2):268-275. Doi: 10.1159/000445883. http://www.ncbi.nlm.nih.gov/pubmed/ 27489560; and ED Goris, KN Ansel, and DL Schutte (2016) "Quantitative Systematic Review of the Effects of Non-pharmacological Interventions on Reducing Apathy in Persons with Dementia." *Journal of Advanced Nursing.* May 25 doi: 10.1111/jan.13026. http://www.ncbi.nlm.nih.gov/pubmed/27221007. Accessed 9/12/2016.

332 MUSIC & MEMORY℠ "MUSIC & MEMORY℠ Helps Wisconsin Nursing Homes Reduce Antipsychotic Use." https://musicandmemory.org/blog/2014/11/14/music-memory%E2%84%A0-helps-wisconsin-nursing-homes-reduce-antipsychotic-use/ Accessed 12/6/2016.

333 MUSIC & MEMORY℠ founded by Dan Cohen. http://musicandmemory.org/. Accessed 9/12/2016. Michael Rossato-Bennett, Director, *Alive Inside* (Alive Inside, LLC, 2014) DVD documentary.

334 MUSIC & MEMORY℠, "Painting Red Trees: How Art Therapy Plus MUSIC & MEMORY℠ Unlocks Advanced Dementia." http://musicandmemory.org/blog/ 2016/04/06/art-therapy-plus-music-memory-unlocks-advanced-dementia/. Accessed 9/12/2016.

335 Department of Health Services, State of Wisconsin, "Instructions to Complete the Power of Attorney for Health Care Form." https://www.dhs.wisconsin.gov/forms/ advdirectives/f00085.pdf. Accessed 9/23/2017. For example, the instructions for completing Wisconsin's Health Care POA, includes the state statutes for activation. You can see a sample of a Power of Attorney for Health Care Statement of Incapacity at https://iconnect.aurora.org/ahcweb3/forms/Forms/x20558-poa-activating-deactivating.pdf. Accessed 12/6/2016.

336 Life Legal Defense Foundation, "POLST: When "Doctor's Orders" Mean Death. https://lifelegaldefensefoundation.org/2014/07/01/polst-when-doctors-orders-mean-death/. Accessed 8/22/2016.

337 K Alagiakrishnan, RA Bhanji, and M Kurian (2013). "Evaluation and management of oropharyngeal dysphagia in different types of dementia: a systematic review." *Archives of Gerontology and Geriatrics* 56(1):1-9 doi:

10.1016/j.archger.2012.04.011. www.ncbi.nlm.nih.gov/pubmed/22608838. Accessed 11/17/2016.

[338] American Geriatrics Society Ethics Committee and Clinical Practice and Models of Care Committee (2014). "American Geriatrics Society Feeding Tubes in Advanced Dementia Position Statement." *Journal of the American Geriatrics Society* 62:1590-1593. https://www.ncbi.nlm.nih.gov/pubmed/25039796. Accessed 9/232017.

[339] Z Mehta, MD; K Giorgini, DO; N Ellison, MD; and ME Roth, MD, FACPE (2012). "Integrating Palliative Medicine with Dementia Care." *Aging Well*, Vol. 5: No. 2, p 18. http://www.todaysgeriatricmedicine.com/archive/031912p18.shtml. Accessed 8/18/2016.

[340] Cummings, pp 311-312; Whitworth and Whitworth, p 213; and Maribeth Gallagher, DNP, PMHNP-BC, FAAN and Jeannette Castellane "Chapter 18. Final Choices: Successfully Navigating Challenges in Advanced and End-of-Life Care" in Gary Radin and Lisa Radin (eds.), *What If It's Not Alzheimer's?: A Caregiver's Guide to Dementia, 3rd ed.* (Amherst, NY: Prometheus Books, 2014), p 294.

[341] Deborah Howard, RN, CHPN, *Sunsets: Reflections for Life's Final Journey* (Wheaton, IL: Crossway, a publishing ministry of Good New Publishers, 2005), p 240.

[342] Gallagher and Castellane, in Radin and Radin, p 291.

[343] Jan Zimmerman, RN, Nursing Administrator, Heritage Homes, Watertown, WI. Interview 5/20/2014.

[344] The Association for Frontotemporal Degeneration, "Comfort Care and Hospice in Advanced FTD." *Partners in FTD Care* Fall 2016. www.theaftd.org/wp-content/ uploads/2016/12/PinFTDcare_Newsletter_Fall_2016.pdf. Accessed 12/9/2016.

[345] Mehta, et al.

[346] Ibid.

[347] Howard, p 168.

[348] Ibid., p 169.

[349] Ibid.

[350] Ibid., p 171.

[351] Ibid., p 176.

[352] Ibid., p 178.

[353] Ibid.

[354] Delving further into the question of euthanasia (bringing on a good death) is beyond the scope of this book.

[355] Dr. Benjamin Mast, *Second Forgetting: Remembering the Power of the Gospel During Alzheimer's Disease* (Grand Rapids, MI: Zondervan, 2014), pp 166-167.

Acknowledgments

M any thanks to God for all the encouragement, support, and help I received during this journey. First, to my husband, Ralph Gable, who allowed me the space to write, encouraged when I lagged, and provided his formatting talents with the book including the cover art. I greatly appreciated the patient guidance of my editors who taught me a great deal over the months. My beta readers were instrumental in tightening the work. I cannot forget to mention my friends at Emmaus International who helped with title suggestions, polishing of the cover design, digital marketing, and designs, as well as the WestBow Press teams.

While many hours must be spent alone, no work develops without the input of many voices. Besides my own experience with my mother, I am deeply grateful for other caregivers willing to share their stories, my Bible study friends willing to help me work through some of the theological issues, and those who answered my questions.

My call to write this book became my need. The Lord continually provided the right help at the right time. God's glory shines through the darkest valleys.

Appendix

Dementia Resources

Good Books

Dunlop, John, MD. *Finding Grace in the Face of Dementia*. Wheaton, IL: Crossway, 2017.

Mace, Nancy L, MA, and Peter V Rabins, MD, MPH. *The 36-Hour Day: A Family Guide to Caring for People Who Have Alzheimer's Disease, Related Dementias, and Memory Loss, 5th ed*. New York: Grand Central Life & Style, 2012.

McQuilkin, Robertson. *A Promise Kept*. Carol Stream, IL: Tyndale House Publishers, Inc., 2006.

Swinton, John. *Dementia: Living in the Memories of God*. Grand Rapids, MI: William B Eerdmans Publishing Company, 2012.

Helpful Organizations & Websites

Dementia Care Central. www.dementiacarecentral.com.

Dementia Society of America. www.dementiasociety.org.

Family Caregiver Alliance. www.caregiver.org.

National Institute on Aging—search on *dementia*. www.nia.nih.gov/

Alzheimer's Disease Resources

Since many with dementia will have some Alzheimer's symptoms, resources written for Alzheimer's will also be helpful for a loved one with another diagnosis.

Good Books

Angelica, Jade C. *Where Two Worlds Touch: A Spiritual Journey through Alzheimer's Disease.* Boston: Skinner House Books, 2014.

Cummings, Tam, PhD. *Untangling Alzheimer's: The Guide for Families and Professionals (A Conversation in Caregiving),* 2nd ed. North Charleston, SC: The Dementia Association LLC, 2015.

Doraiswamy, P Murali, MD, and Lisa P Gwyther, MSW, with Tina Adler. *The Alzheimer's Action Plan: What You Need to Know— What You Can Do—about Memory Problems, from Prevention to Early Intervention and Care.* New York: St. Martin's Press, 2008.

McLay, Evelyn and Ellen P Young. *Mom's OK, She Just Forgets: The Alzheimer's Journey from Denial to Acceptance.* Amherst, NY: Prometheus Books, 2006.

Newport, Mary, MD. *Alzheimer's Disease: What If There Was a Cure? The Story of Ketones,* 2nd ed. Laguna Beach, CA: Basic Health Publications, Inc., 2013.

Pearce, Nancy D. *Inside Alzheimer's: How to Hear and Honor Connections with a Person who has Dementia.* Taylors, SC: Forrason Press, 2007.

Petersen, Ronald, MD, PhD. *Mayo Clinic Guide to Alzheimer's Disease.* Rochester, MN: Mayo Clinic, 2006.

Shanks, Lela Knox. *Your Name Is Hughes Hannibal Shanks: A Caregiver's Guide to Alzheimer's.* Lincoln, NE: University of Nebraska Press, 1999.

Zeisel, John, PhD. *I'm Still Here: A New Philosophy of Alzheimer's Care.* New York: Avery: Penguin Group USA, 2010.

Alzheimer's association. www.alz.org. Various states and countries have their own Alzheimer's sites with useful information.

Alzheimer's Reading Room. www.alzheimersreadingroom.com.

National Institute on Aging has its own portal for Alzheimer's resources. www.alzheimers.gov.

Frontotemporal Dementia Resources

Good Book

Radin, Gary and Lisa, editors. *What If It's Not Alzheimer's?:A Caregiver's Guide to Dementia*, 3rd ed. Amherst, NY: Prometheus Books, 2014.

Helpful Organization & Website

The Association for Frontotemporal Degeneration. www.theaftd.org.

Lewy Body Dementia Resources

Good Books

Towne Jennings, Judy, PT, MA. *Living with Lewy Body Dementia: One Caregiver's Personal, In-Depth Experience*. Bloomington, IN: WestBow Press, a Division of Thomas Nelson, 2012.

Whitworth, Helen Buell and James. *A Caregiver's Guide to Lewy Body Dementia*. New York: demosHealth, 2011.

Helpful Organization & Website

Lewy Body Dementia Association. www.lbda.org.

Other Helpful Resources

Amador, Xavier, Ph.D. *I Am Not Sick, I Don't Need Help! How to Help Someone with Mental Illness Accept Treatment.* 10th Anniversary Edition. New York: Vida Press, 2012.

Bramsen, Nate. *What If Jesus Meant What He Said?* Dubuque, IA: Emmaus International, 2017.

Eareckson Tada, Joni. *A Place of Healing: Wrestling with the Mysteries of Suffering, Pain, and God's Sovereignty.* USA: David C. Cook, 2010.

Eareckson Tada, Joni. *When Is It Right to Die? A Comforting and Surprising Look at Death and Dying: An Updated Edition.* Grand Rapids, MI: Zondervan Publishing House, a Division of Harper Collins Publishers, 2018

Hernandez, Amy. *Unstuck: Moving Beyond Defeat.* Dubuque, IA: Emmaus International, 2015.

Howard, Deborah, RN, CHPN. *Sunsets: Reflections for Life's Final Journey.* Wheaton, IL: Crossway, a publishing ministry of Good New Publishers, 2005.

Keller, Timothy. *Walking with God through Pain and Suffering.* New York: Riverhead Books, An imprint of Penguin Random House, LLC, 2015.

McQuilkin, Robertson and Paul Copan. *An Introduction to Biblical Ethics: Walking in the Way of Wisdom, Third Edition.* Downers Grove,IL: IVP Academic, An imprint of InterVarsity Press, 2014.

Index

Printed in the United States
By Bookmasters